W9-BTG-805

Diet for a Pain-Free Life
WILL CHANGE YOUR LIFE...

"When my pain medication was suddenly withdrawn by the FDA, I didn't know what to do. So I started *Diet for a Pain-Free Life* out of desperation to end my knee pain. When I quickly dropped 10 pounds without feeling hungry, I was thrilled. Losing 10 pounds was the answer for me. My pain is gone most days, and I no longer take any medication."
—Paul, age 55

"After one week on the Pain-Free Diet, I lost 8½ pounds. My fasting blood glucose went from 190 to 122, and I was walking without any pain. I was thrilled and so was my primary care doctor. This is definitely a diet for life—my life!"
—Frank, age 66

"For years my back pain dominated my life. I missed so many family activities because of the nagging tenderness and fatigue. Now I've lost 23 pounds and feel years younger. I can do anything—ride bikes with my son, go dancing with my husband, and even join my teenage daughter at a low-impact aerobics class. What's so great is that I seem to eat all day long but the pounds continue to drop. Life is so good!"
—Sarah, age 46

"When I was diagnosed with fibromyalgia with the deep muscle pain, I thought I was destined to a life of lying on the couch, watching cable news all day. Then I started *Diet for a Pain-Free Life*. The diet helped me to lose 18 pounds, and I'm delighted. I am active now and sleep 7 hours a night. This program gave me back my independence and also helped to control my pain."
—Maria, age 38

"After years of being overweight and living daily with lower back and knee pain, I was desperate to find relief. I had even considered stomach bypass surgery until Dr. McIlwain asked me to try the Pain-Free Diet at a routine visit last year. Admittedly, I'm a meat eater and the idea of eliminating all beef, pork, and veal from my diet was not attractive.

But I was tired of being fat and limited in my daily activities, so I decided to give it a try. My partner and I found some delicious 'fake meat' alternatives at the supermarket, and we created new dishes that were incredible. Within 21 days, I had dropped 6 pounds and my knees and back were not as achy when I got up in the morning. After four months, I had lost 26 pounds and was riding a stationary bike for an hour most days—and I had no pain at all. I'll admit that I've never felt this healthy or been this active, and I eat all day long."

—Warren, age 52

"I was diagnosed with osteoarthritis of the spine in my early 40s and have suffered with chronic back pain ever since. While I used to play tennis and swim when my kids were young, the constant back pain kept me from doing much else except for working each day. I was fat, 50, and unfit—and had virtually lost interest in life. I started the Pain-Free Diet right after the super aspirins were taken off the market by the FDA. I was hopeful that the diet might work to ease my pain but I didn't realize how much my entire life would change. Since starting the diet and the other three steps, I've lost 14 pounds. I swim laps each morning at the local Y, and am dating a wonderful man who I met at my water aerobics class. Every pain sufferer should be on the Pain-Free Diet; every baby boomer should use this 4-step program to reignite their lives."

—Jillian, age 54

"After watching my wife drop 12 pounds in two months on the Pain-Free Diet, I decided to try it myself. Now we have lost a total of 41 pounds and are considered slightly overweight instead of obese. The biggest difference we've seen is in our energy level, which is high most days, and in our ability to do anything we want without feeling pain, including exercise, gardening, and recreational sports. Last summer we traveled to Europe with a group of friends and went on several biking tours in England. We could have never done this when we were so heavy—and hurting. This diet gave us an active retirement and we are thrilled!"

—Thomas, age 67

Diet
for a
Pain-Free
Life

A Revolutionary Plan to Lose Weight,
Stop Pain, Sleep Better
and Feel Great in 21 Days

Harris H. McIlwain, MD
and Debra Fulghum Bruce, PhD

MARLOWE & COMPANY
NEW YORK

DIET FOR A PAIN-FREE LIFE:
A Revolutionary Plan to Lose Weight,
Stop Pain, Sleep Better and Feel Great in 21 Days

Copyright © 2006 by Harris H. McIlwain, MD and Debra Fulghum Bruce, PhD
Illustrations copyright © 2006 by James Russell, MS

Published by
Marlowe & Company
An Imprint of Avalon Publishing Group, Incorporated
245 West 17th Street • 11th Floor
New York, NY 10011-5300

AVALON
publishing group incorporated

Library of Congress Cataloging-in-Publication Data is available

ISBN-10: 1-56924-269-0
ISBN-13: 978-1-56924-269-8

9 8 7 6 5 4 3 2 1

DESIGNED BY PAULINE NEUWIRTH, NEUWIRTH & ASSOCIATES, INC.

Printed in the United States of America

To the millions of baby boomers who suffer with chronic pain. May they find new hope and help with this 4-step program to reduce weight, inflammation, and pain, and rediscover what it means to be active and alive once again!

Contents

Preface

T ENS OF MILLIONS of Americans live with pain on a daily basis. Many are overweight. And for most of these individuals, they felt fine until they hit middle age.

As a pain specialist with one of the largest rheumatology group practices in the South, I passionately believe that chronic pain is a pandemic lifestyle disease. Harmful habits such as a fast-food diet, lack of exercise, chronic stress, and poor sleep make us highly susceptible to long-term pain that perpetuates itself. The larger concern I address in this book is America's obesity epidemic—specifically, how extra fat, particularly belly fat, triggers low-grade inflammation in the body, which results in pain and serious illness.

For the past twenty-five years, I have focused on the connection between overweight, inflammation, and chronic pain, and have identified a revolutionary 4-step program that can reverse this deleterious process in most people. That program is the Diet for a Pain-Free Life, hereafter called Pain-Free Diet for short.

As a board-certified rheumatologist, adjunct professor in the College of Public Health at the University of South Florida, and investigator in clinical trials at Tampa Medical Group Research, over the past three decades I have seen thousands of men and women who have suffered with chronic pain from back or neck problems, arthritis, fibromyalgia, and sports injuries, and other conditions. Early in my career, I watched the most physically active men and women become inactive and even dependent on caregivers as they moved into their forties, fifties, and sixties and lived with the results of ignoring their weight—which greatly burdened their muscles, joints, and bones, and impacted their ability to be active. Many of my patients were star athletes in high school and college. Others thrived on active weekends, engaging in recreational and competitive sports or active gardening. Yet, in an almost predictable way, as these overweight baby boomer men and women hit middle age, they would come to my office asking for strong medications to end their chronic (long-term) joint and muscle pain and stiffness so they could do the activities they enjoyed. According to the Centers for Disease Control, obesity has roughly the same association with chronic health conditions as twenty years of aging. Obese and overweight men and women spend 3.5 times more on prescription drugs than those who are normal weight

Predicting the tremendous impact of chronic pain on the millions of aging baby boomers, in 1999, some renowned pharmaceutical giants released "super aspirins." These medications targeted inflammation, the living tissue response to mechanical, chemical, and immunological challenge, and allowed patients to be active again—virtually without pain. Many of my patients participated in the clinical trials for these super aspirins at Tampa Medical Group Research and were thrilled with the results. They were once again able to enjoy recreational sports and other activities.

Then in September 2004, we all awoke to learn that the manufacturer of the arthritis drug Vioxx voluntarily removed the product from the market. This was after a large cancer-prevention study found an increased risk of heart attack and stroke in study participants treated with Vioxx (compared to those treated with placebo). Likewise, the popular pain reliever Bextra was removed just a short time later for similar concerns. In all, removal of these key boomer medications left more than *100 million people worldwide* who had taken super aspirins without adequate treatment for pain-related problems. I vividly remember the day when this occurred, as hundreds of patients called my clinic, clamoring for an alternative to the super aspirins that had miraculously given them pain-free lives and allowed them to be active.

The reality is that aging is inevitable; no one is immune. There is no miracle cure. It's true that aging can increase the release of destructive, proinflammatory chemicals in the body, which in turn can increase chronic pain, but we now know that carrying extra weight triggers the same proinflammatory chemicals. Although we cannot stop aging, we *can* lose weight to significantly decrease the low-grade inflammation and resulting pain.

From the thousands of patients I have treated since 1980, along with the major discoveries in the field of pain medicine, I concluded that almost all of my pain patients could benefit from a plant-based diet filled with antiinflammatory foods. I have recommended this Pain-Free Diet to many patients over the years and the results have been phenomenal, as I describe in this book.

Since I started my practice, I have learned so much more about the human body and how to keep patients in optimal health and living active, productive lives. Throughout this book, I want to help you understand the important connection between excess weight (particularly belly fat), inflammation, and pain, and I'll teach you surefire ways to start reversing the cycle now. I want you and your family to see how anti-inflammatory foods can boost weight loss, whereas pro-inflammatory foods can increase pounds—and pain. Above all, I want to help you live each day feeling energetic and be as active as you'd like to be. With the 4-step program in *Diet for a Pain-Free Life*, I know you'll be feeling pain free soon.

Start today. You can protect your health and the health of your family. I hope this book will provide you with the tools you will need to determine a safe and balanced roadmap to losing weight and ending pain—once and for all.

—HARRIS H. MCILWAIN, MD
August 2006

Getting Started:
What You Must Know to Live Pain Free

Y OU LOOK IN the mirror as you get ready for bed and see a heavy, older person peering back at you. Who is that overweight person? Admittedly, you're not as thin and fit as you used to be ... after all, you're not in your twenties, and this added girth goes with the territory, right? Still, you wish your waistline hadn't expanded quite so much.

While the extra pounds bother you, what you really wish you could control is the pain. It's there 24/7—from your aching lower back that keeps you from sleeping well at night, to the knee pain that forced you to give up tennis. Then there is the nagging twinge in your right hip that even medication cannot stop.

"Lose weight," says your physician. *But how?* you think to yourself. You've never been able to stay on a diet. Then you worry that maybe your doctor is right. If you don't lose some weight, you're a sure candidate for reparative or replacement surgery. But the idea of undergoing surgery seems so risky; after all, there's general anesthesia, time off from work, and months of recovery, not to mention the cost. . . . Didn't your co-worker have some awful side effects from back surgery recently? What about your cousin who had the hip replacement and still has tremendous pain?

Sighing, you finish getting ready for bed and lie awake for what seems like hours trying to get comfortable. The next day, despite your best intentions, you forgo the morning exercise regimen your doctor prescribed. Instead, you sit in your cubicle at work, sipping colas and snacking on cheese crackers from the vending machine, and then rush home with some cheeseburgers and fries for a quick meal with the kids before crashing in your recliner . . . and getting up the next day just to do it all again.

If you suffer from daily pain, you're not alone. As many as 150 million Americans live with chronic pain. This includes 45 million people who suffer with the constant pain of *arthritis* (*rheumatoid* arthritis and *osteoarthritis*), 15 million who live with the deep muscle pain and fatigue of *fibromyalgia syndrome*, and at least four out of five Americans who suffer with neck or back pain, whether from a sports injury, poor muscle tone, or disk disease. The pain statistics don't end there. Millions more Americans live with the daily pain and stiffness of *carpal tunnel syndrome*, shoulder pain, *tendinitis*, *bursitis*, and chronic pain resulting from recreational or sports injuries.

No matter what type of pain you have, you know how pain can affect all aspects of life—your marital and family relationships, productivity and ability to earn a living, sleep, eating habits, and overall health. Pain can even stop you from enjoying life's pleasures, from traveling on vacation to even hugging your child or grandchild.

Identify Your Pain Problems

NO MATTER WHICH pain problems you have, you will find tremendous relief with this 4-step program. Check the pain problems that bother you most.

- ❏ Osteoarthritis ("wear and tear" arthritis)
- ❏ Back pain
- ❏ Neck pain
- ❏ Sore muscles
- ❏ Fibromyalgia (deep muscle pain)
- ❏ Inflamed joints
- ❏ Rheumatoid arthritis (and other inflammatory types)
- ❏ Stiffness
- ❏ Sleep problems
- ❏ Hip pain
- ❏ Knee pain

❏ Shoulder pain
❏ Ankle pain
❏ Tennis elbow
❏ Disk disease
❏ Fatigue
❏ Weak muscles
❏ Pain and stiffness after exercise
❏ Poor sleep because of pain

WHEN PAIN BECOMES THE DISEASE

It may seem surprising to some that pain is still a critical battle in our technically sophisticated society, with all the health advancements and medical breakthroughs—but it is. That's because pain is a basic physiological response—a warning sign in your body that lets you know something is wrong.

Our understanding of the body's pain mechanism stems from decades of research studies. One of the most important was Dr. Ronald Melzack and Dr. Patrick Wall's "gate control theory," which was published in 1965. This theory suggests that there is a "gating system" in the central nervous system that opens and closes, either to let pain messages into the brain or to block them. The basis for the theory is the belief that psychological as well as physical factors channel the brain's understanding of painful feelings and the ensuing response.

I know it is difficult to think of pain as a positive sign, but it is. Pain is a vital, protective mechanism that signals there is a potential problem. Without this warning, you might cause irreparable injury to the body.

But while this feeling is the body's way of alerting the brain that there is a problem, after going on for weeks to months, pain can become a part of your entire existence. At that point, not only is pain a symptom that something is amiss, but pain becomes the disease *itself*. Let me explain.

Acute or Chronic?

Pain falls into one of two categories: *acute* or *chronic*. Acute pain comes on suddenly and can be severe. For instance, if you live with constant back pain, you know how quickly your back can ache after you bend down to pick up a heavy package. Findings show that more than 70 percent of Americans have acute pain from headache at some time each year; over 50 percent have back-aches. Yet, in more than 80 percent of cases, acute pain goes away in about two weeks; it runs its course and disappears as the problem is relieved.

When acute pain lasts for weeks into months then it is called chronic pain, and the body begins to behave differently. Chronic pain prevents sleep and often results in daytime fatigue, poor concentration, irritability, and difficulty dealing with others, including family members, friends, and co-workers. For those who juggle caregiving with careers, chronic pain can make life seem overwhelming with feelings of anxiety, anger, depression, hopelessness, and even suicide.

Chronic pain is relentless—and expensive, with social costs in disability and lost productivity estimated at more than $100 billion annually. Chronic pain causes nearly 40 million visits to doctors and other health-care providers and can extend hospital stays, hinder recovery, and intensely change your quality of life.

Chronic pain is also unhealthy. Unlike acute pain, which is a sign of a healthy nervous system, chronic pain takes on its own life and mimics a disease. When pain persists for weeks or even months, it can cause an increase in the level of *cortisol*, the body's main stress-induced hormone. Although the immune system needs a certain amount of cortisol, when it becomes elevated for an extended period, it can impair the cells that make up your immune system and kidney function.

When bathed in this stress-related chemical, the immune system can find it harder to function optionally. Living with unending chronic pain and the subsequent stress, your immune system simply will not work at full capacity. This breakdown in immune function can interfere with your ability to fight infections, your long-term healing, and your overall quality of life. In fact, there are new studies that indicate pain may affect the immune system in such a way that cancer cells speed up their growth when there is pain in the body.

What Is Inflammation— And What Does That Have to Do with Your Pain?

Since pain is a sign that something is amiss in the body, it's important to understand how pain is linked to *inflammation*, to comprehend how *Diet for a Pain-Free Life* can help you.

Here's how it works: inflammation is the body's immune system response to fight infections and other outside "invaders." White blood cells, part of the body's defense, create proteins and other compounds to eliminate infections and protect the body. In addition, when the body's immune system detects foreign proteins, the immune system can react to eliminate that "invader." Normally only foreign bacteria, viruses, and abnormal cells are the targets for this immune reaction.

But sometimes, the immune system creates inflammation that attacks the body's own tissues. In other words, the body turns against itself, resulting in serious illness, such as arthritis with joint pain and swelling and inflammation in other areas including the kidneys, heart, skin, and other organs. Research shows that inflammation is a key factor in such diseases as heart disease, stroke, and diabetes, among others.

How Do You Feel Pain?

Your body has roughly twenty different nerve endings in the skin that tell you if something is hot, cold, or going to be painful. The nerve endings convey this information to the brain and spinal cord, also known as the central nervous system, areas where we perceive the stimuli. To accomplish this, the nerve endings of the sensory receptors convert mechanical, thermal, or chemical energy into electrical signals or the painful sensations you actually feel: searing, burning, pounding, or throbbing, among others.

However, pain is more than what you feel at a particular anatomical site. Researchers believe that pain is in your nerves. When pain is chronic or long-term, not only do you hurt, but you also may experience:

- Insomnia
- Daytime sleepiness
- Irritability
- Difficulty concentrating
- Appetite loss or increase
- Muscle weakness
- Low energy
- Depression

All of these can make it difficult, if not impossible, to do your daily tasks, including caring for your family and working outside the home. That's why we must look at pain, the various causes, and how it can be resolved differently . . . instead of relying on a "magic pill." Moreover, at this writing, we know that there is no magic pill.

Going beyond Medications

Maybe you depend on several *over-the-counter (OTC) medications* each day to get adequate relief from your pain. Or perhaps you need stronger prescription pain medications but live with the undesirable side effects of fatigue, irritability, and an inability to concentrate at work.

As a medical doctor and board-certified *rheumatologist*, I diagnose and treat pain-related problems daily. Do I ever prescribe pain medications? Of course. I am passionate about finding new medical breakthroughs to help my patients ease the signs and symptoms of pain and debilitating illnesses such as arthritis, back pain, and fibromyalgia. I have done clinical trials on an array of experimental medications for more than two decades, hoping to identify those drugs that give the best relief. While I have found some medications that offer good relief of long-term pain, others have not been as helpful because of unwanted side effects. For example, to get some relief from inflammation and pain, more than 34 million Americans use various *nonsteroidal anti-inflammatory drugs (NSAIDs)* on a daily basis. Yet these medications have side effects that can be serious—even deadly. In fact, some new findings indicate that high doses of traditional NSAIDs can raise the risk of heart attack. When two of the most potent *anti-inflammatory* pain relievers—Vioxx and Bextra—were removed from the market in 2004, millions of men and women were left without adequate relief.

So where *do* you turn for relief? How many times have you caught fragments of a news report about a revolutionary new medication that *may* help end chronic pain, or a cutting-edge surgical procedure that *may* reduce excruciating pain? Perhaps you were impressed at the innovations of modern medicine and could not wait to learn more.

Although today's medicine is changing at incredible speed, allowing doctors to diagnose and treat pain-related problems in the earliest stages when treatment is more effective, there is powerful scientific evidence that we have completely ignored the *very best* treatment for preventing and reversing pain.

WEIGHT LOSS IS THE SECRET

As pain specialists with three large clinics on Florida's Gulf Coast, my partners and I see hundreds of patients each week. Although our patients participate in a variety of clinical trials, helping to find a better medication for pain, I have found there is a simpler solution. *Diet for a Pain-Free Life* is the first book ever to illustrate how weight loss of as little as 10 pounds—along with an anti-inflammatory diet—can reverse the cycle of chronic pain. This method results in extraordinary cellular changes at a microscopic level in the body that decrease low-grade inflammation, resulting in less pain, stiffness and disability.

Simply stated, the more overweight you are, the greater the level of pro-inflammatory markers in your body and the greater your risk of pain. For example, during episodes of acute inflammation, your liver produces a special type of protein called *C-reactive protein (CRP)*. This protein is highly associated with obesity, cardiovascular disease, diabetes, and cancer. In addition, some groundbreaking findings now indicate that there are elevated levels of C-reactive protein in patients with inflammatory arthritis, *osteoarthritis*, and other pain-related ailments. (There are other pro-inflammatory markers produced by the body, which I will discuss later in the book.)

Thousands of my patients have successfully adopted the *Diet for a Pain-Free Life* 4-step lifestyle plan, and lost 10 to 50 pounds or even more. Many of my patients saw weight loss of 5 to 8 pounds or more after just 21 days. And, in almost every one of my patients, the weight loss was directly correlated with a significant decrease of pro-inflammatory markers (like C-reactive protein), as well as a decrease in LDL ("bad") cholesterol and triglyceride levels, blood pressure, fasting blood glucose levels, and, best of all, a decrease in both frequency and intensity of chronic joint and muscle pain.

Is the Pain-Free Diet for You?

Imagine that you are wearing a coat that weighs 10, 20, or 30 pounds. Think about how this heavy coat affects every part of your life—from the way you walk, sit, and sleep to how you function in daily activities at home and in the workplace.

Now envision taking off this imaginary coat. Feel the tremendous relief your body must feel without the added weight on your joints, muscles, and heart. This is what this program has done for my patients—and it can do the same for you. No matter what you weigh now, no matter how high the degree of your pain, you *can* live an active, pain-free life!

• • •

Stopping a Diabetes Epidemic

ACCORDING TO DATA from the National Health and Nutrition Examination Survey (NHANES), more than 1 in every 3 Americans have diabetes. Researchers estimate that one-third of diabetics are undiagnosed and do not know they have it. The four steps in the Pain-Free Diet can greatly reduce your risk of diabetes as well as end your battle with pain.

Beverly Reclaims Her Active Life

Let's take my patient Beverly, as an example. Beverly, age 55, is a successful real estate broker who thrives on being active. Married for thirty-five years, she and her husband raised four children and are now renovating a sprawling estate near the Gulf of Mexico right outside of Tampa, Florida. About fifteen years ago, Beverly fell going down a flight of stairs and injured her back. She went through physical therapy and continued to do the recommended back exercises for a while, but as with most of us, the busy-ness of life took over, and Beverly had little time to focus on herself. What she gained in extra time in her early forties, she paid for in her early fifties with increased weight, back pain, and an inability to be active.

Each time I saw Beverly over the past decade, I'd suggest that she might change some lifestyle habits and follow my Pain-Free Diet to lose weight, manage her stress, improve her sleep, and exercise properly to resolve her back pain. Beverly would always admit she just did not have time to watch what she ate or exercise and would leave my office by saying, "Maybe this time I will get serious about my back pain."

Several times during this period, Beverly would tell of going on a very-low-fat, high carbohydrate diet. No matter how strictly she followed the plan, she would end up gaining 10 to 15 pounds instead of losing the weight. We now know that low-fat/high-carbohydrate diets increase the level of fat in the blood and lower high-density lipoprotein cholesterol (HDL, or "good") cholesterol of some people, *particularly women over forty*, and cause an *increase* in weight instead of weight loss. In fact, in people who are insulin resistant, a diet high in carbohydrates such as pasta and white potatoes activates enzymes involved in fat storage. Currently 50 million Americans—mostly baby boomers—suffer from metabolic syndrome and have risk factors such as type 2 diabetes, hypertension, high triglycerides, and low HDL cholesterol. Obesity and insulin resistance are also signs of metabolic syndrome.

As time went by, Beverly's pain increased so much she had difficulty sleeping. On a scale of 1 to 10, she rated her pain at 9 most days. She told me she would finally get up and read about 3:00 AM, because she could not get comfortable in bed. She would then pay deeply for this the next day, as it would be difficult to be productive and alert on the job. Beverly was also unable to attend her daughter's graduation from dental school because she could not tolerate the three-hour drive in a car. But when her first grandchildren—twin boys—were born and Beverly could not pick them up, she realized that her back pain had taken over her life.

"When I saw these beautiful babies and I knew I could not lift them, I cried," she remembers. "I was so distressed that my back pain controlled every part of my life. I was angry that it directed what I did each day, where I went, and how active I could be. But this time, I was ready to fight my pain.

"The next morning, I called the dietitian you had recommended, and together we went over your Pain-Free Diet. She showed me how to include legumes, soy products, and fish in my diet as a substitute for meat. I went from eating one fruit each day to three or four, and I have not been hungry at all.

"I joined a fitness center near our home, and signed up for water aerobics and a stretching class. Since that time, I have spent every day of the last seven months working on changing the way I eat, adding some key nutrients with dietary supplements, strengthening my muscles with weight training, learning how to manage my daily stress, and improving my sleep quality. I am finally committed to taking charge of my life—and pain.

"I've now lost 32 pounds, even though I seem to eat all day long. I swim and ride bikes daily, and my back pain is almost completely gone. I am shocked that such simple steps as eating differently, losing weight, and moving around more gave me total control of my life again."

Beverly is just one of thousands of people who have witnessed the dramatic change that can happen when you take charge of your pain—instead of allowing it to dominate your life. And like so many of my patients have experienced with great success, it all starts with small changes, one day at a time—adjusting the foods you eat, and altering your stress response and your exercise and sleep habits.

Weight Loss Results in a Pain-Free Life

The Pain-Free Diet is not a quick fix for years of ignoring your weight. In fact, there are other fad diets that may enable you to drop weight faster and see results more quickly. But as a physician, I'll tell you up front that these fad diets also set you up for rapid weight gain when you no longer can adhere to the rigid rules such as only eating foods that are very low calorie, very low fat, or very low in carbohydrates. You need to allow a few weeks (Level 1, called Jump Start) to change a lifetime of poor eating habits as you eliminate most animal foods (particularly beef, pork, and veal) from your diet, along with processed and packaged foods like chips, cookies, crackers, and sweetened cereals and fast foods (french fries, shakes, and onion rings).

After staying on the Pain-Free Diet for 21 days, you will feel lighter, healthier, less pain. At two months on the program, your clothes will be a size too big, you will feel energetic, and your chronic pain will be dramatically reduced so you feel like being more active with exercise. At six months on the Pain-Free Diet, you will probably feel better than you've felt in years—maybe even decades—and will probably be able to be as active as you want without the interruption of nagging pain. Once you've lost the unwanted pounds, I highly recommend that you stay on the Pain-Free Diet for a lifetime, adding more foods and calories to maintain your goal weight. After all, once you live pain free, you'll never want to return to a life of pain and limitation.

In the past twenty-five years of clinical practice, I've had patients who had tried every weight-loss diet available finally agree to try the Pain-Free Diet and effortlessly lose 15 pounds in three months or less. While this may not seem dramatic to some people who want to see immediate results, this weight loss literally gave them back their lives. Instead of being sedentary, they were able to walk on a treadmill each day, walk their dog around the neighborhood after work, and enjoy recreational activities with family and friends. Because they weighed less, they no longer hurt during exercise, which increased their desire and ability to be more active. As they followed Rx #1 of the diet for three months, six months, and then a year, not only did they drop most of the excess weight, but they found their pain was greatly reduced (or even resolved for many patients) and their quality of life greatly increased. Most importantly from a medical standpoint, their blood pressure and cholesterol levels normalized, as did the blood levels of pro-inflammatory markers in their body.

UNDERSTANDING THE
OBESITY-INFLAMMATION-PAIN CONNECTION

Joseph's Obesity and Knee Pain

I have treated Joseph since he first came to our clinic about fifteen years ago with complaints of knee pain. At the time, this 5'11" chemistry teacher and part-time high school soccer coach was slightly overweight at 190 pounds. Now in his midfifties, Joseph has an administrative position with the county school board. He no longer plays soccer and, at a visit to my office one year ago, he tipped the scale at 230 pounds. "Lately when I walk to the parking lot or bend down to pick up something off the floor, the knee pain takes my breath away," Joseph said. "I sometimes hesitate in going out with my kids or colleagues for fear the pain will be more than I can bear."

When I calculated his *body mass index* (BMI, a key indicator for relating body weight to height, Joseph was in the "obese" range. Not only does a higher BMI put someone at a greater risk of developing heart disease, cancer, or diabetes, it signifies the presence of inflammation in the body, which is a key trigger of pain. (I will explain how to determine your BMI on page 68.)

Obesity represents a state of excess storage of body fat and is epidemic in the United States with an estimated 110 million adults in the United States (about 65 percent of the population) are clinically overweight or obese with a body mass index higher than 25. Likewise, pain is another extremely common complaint, affecting from 75 to 150 million people in the United States. Researchers have clearly linked obesity and pain with similar pro-inflammatory markers or physiological substances in the blood that indicate disease when present in abnormal amounts. Realizing the tie between excess weight and pain, my partners and I have searched for new therapeutic ways to treat them.

While Joseph thought his excess body fat was simply a problem of aesthetics, I explained that it had a much greater significance than what he could see or feel. Although it is poorly understood, we now know that fatty tissue is a major endocrine organ that produces hormones just like other organs in the body. It secretes influential pro-inflammatory chemicals, messengers that contribute to low-grade inflammation, diseases, and pain.

It is thought that as fat tissue in the body increases, the blood vessels feeding this tissue are not sufficient to maintain a normal oxygen supply and there is a localized reduction of oxygen. This oxygen deprivation triggers pro-inflammatory reactions, which can produce more cell-damaging substances in the body. Obesity can cause this response to go out of control and can add to problems such as pain, diabetes mellitus, hypertension, heart disease and some types of cancer.

In Joseph's case, not only did he suffer from joint pain in his knees, but the lab taken at his last visit revealed that he had high triglycerides, high LDL cholesterol, and low HDL cholesterol. (You want your triglycerides and LDL cholesterol levels to be low; your HDL cholesterol should be high.) Joseph's lab also indicated that he was insulin resistant. Insulin is one of the body's hormones that controls blood glucose. Normally, when the body senses a higher glucose level, insulin is released to lower the level of glucose. But with insulin resistance, the body steadily becomes less responsive to the actions of insulin. Despite the high levels of insulin, the blood sugar levels rise, and eventually type 2 diabetes results. People who are insulin resistant tend to gain belly fat—with increasing waistlines (the apple shape as opposed to the pear shape). Like Joseph, these individuals also have elevated triglycerides, low HDL cholesterol, high blood pressure, and high blood glucose levels.

Joseph and I had a long talk about his health status and his desire to get in control of his body. Joseph committed to following the Pain-Free Diet and began meeting with our staff dietitian and physical therapist for education and encouragement to stick with the plan. I also started him on a cholesterol-lowering medication. In four months on the Pain-Free Diet and lifestyle plan, Joseph lost 19 pounds and his lab work was now in normal ranges. He said that riding a stationary bike allowed him to exercise twice daily and build stronger muscles without adding more weight to his arthritic joints. Not only did he feel more energetic and positive about life, his pain and increased risk of serious diseases dropped dramatically.

Scientists now suspect that the increase in pro-inflammatory markers plays a big role in most obesity complications, including *joint and muscle pain that will not subside*. In other words, as Joseph and so many patients have experienced, the heavier you are, the higher your levels of pro-inflammatory markers, and the increase in pain, illness, and even disability. When pro-inflammatory markers activate fat cells in the obese person to produce even more pro-inflammatory markers, a vicious cycle of obesity, inflammation, and pain has begun.

More Weight, More Pain

THE HEAVIER YOU are, the greater the pressure on your ankles, knees, and hips. The National Health and Nutrition Examination Survey reported that obese men are five times more likely to develop knee osteoarthritis than are men who are of normal weight. Obese women are four times more likely to get knee osteoporosis than are women of normal weight.

OBESITY ⟹ INFLAMMATION ⟹ PAIN

What Are the "Pro-Inflammatory Markers"?

Cytokines Cause Joint Pain and Cartilage Destruction

Cytokines are a group of compounds that modulate the activities of cells and function as intercellular messengers. Although the actual role of cytokines is still being understood, we know that some cytokines make inflammation progress and are referred to as pro-inflammatory cytokines. As an example, Interleukin-1 (IL-1) and *tumor necrosis factor (TNF)* are both pro-inflammatory cytokines. When these cytokines are administered to humans in research laboratories, they trigger inflammation, fever, tissue destruction, and even shock and death. Cytokines, including histamine, prostaglandins, TNF-alpha, IL-1, and Interlukin-6 (IL-6), can be identified and measured with specific blood tests.

Erin was forty-three when I first diagnosed her with fibromyalgia, a common condition particularly among women that is characterized by deep muscle pain and tenderness, fatigue, anxiety, insomnia, and depression, among other symptoms. This once-active woman was an avid tennis player in her twenties and early thirties, but when the muscle pain and fatigue kicked in around age forty, she could barely swing a racket, much less brush her young daughter's hair. Erin told me that she "hurt all the time." She said even cooking dinner for her family of five triggered pain, so she relied mostly on fast-food take-out dinners. While the highly processed diet may have satisfied her husband and three children, Erin had gained more than 20 pounds in just one year.

As I have seen repeatedly with other patients, Erin's lab was consistent with her weight gain, showing high levels of LDL cholesterol and low levels of HDL cholesterol. Cytokines, which can trigger pain and joint damage, are inflammatory chemicals which are important in many painful disorders such as fibromyalgia, rheumatoid arthritis, osteoarthritis (the "wear and tear" disease), degenerative lumbar spine disorders, and disk-related back pain.

As an example, in rheumatoid or inflammatory arthritis, TNF is overproduced in the joints. Researchers believe that, in this disease, TNF triggers inflammation that results in the destruction of bone and cartilage. This marker also causes the pain, fever, weight loss, and fatigue associated with arthritis. Understanding that TNF may trigger other enzymes in the body, scientists now believe that blocking it can relieve or stop the effects of inflammation.

High levels of pro-inflammatory cytokines have also been found in tissue samples of patients with early osteoarthritis. Osteoarthritis, the most common form of arthritis, affects adults at every age. Yet the prevalence of this painful condition increases dramatically with age with the greatest incidence in subjects over the age of forty. Moreover, *obesity is a key risk factor.* In fact, hip and knee osteoarthritis are both correlated with excess weight and cause the highest rate of disability in obese patients.

Although some newer drugs can regulate cytokines, there is still the concern that suppressing cytokines could have adverse effects on the immune system, such as an increased risk of infections—sinusitis, pneumonia, and other problems. The answer? Focus on other natural therapies that can reverse inflammation—therapies such as switching to a plant-based diet, losing weight, managing your stress, exercising daily, and getting restful sleep.

C-Reactive Protein Increases Pain Severity

Another key pro-inflammatory marker linked to obesity and pain is C-reactive protein (CRP), a special type of protein produced by the liver that is increased in the blood in response to inflammation. People who smoke, have high blood pressure, are overweight, and don't exercise often have elevated levels of C-reactive protein, whereas lean, active people usually have lower levels. And while C-reactive protein is a marker of increased risk of heart disease, some new studies indicate that the severity of pain from many musculoskeletal disorders is directly related to *higher levels* of C-reactive protein.

Take Laurel, as an example. I had treated this thirty-nine-year-old magazine editor for *low back pain* with occasional sciatica (lower back pain that radiates down the leg and into the foot) since her college days at Emory University, when she had slipped on icy pavement while walking across campus. After working in a sedentary job for almost fifteen years, Laurel's weight had gone from 121 pounds at age twenty-four to 149 pounds today. At 5' 2", this excess weight made it difficult for her to be active. But when you combine Laurel's weight with her ongoing back pain, it was a formula for disaster.

At a recent office visit, Laurel said she had read about there being a connection between high levels of C-reactive protein and pain and obesity, and asked if we would check her blood levels. When Laurel's lab came back, her CRP level *was* elevated. Laurel and I talked openly about her weight and the back pain that could not be resolved, linking these two problems to serious diseases she might face in the future, such as heart disease or diabetes.

Because Laurel (like so many patients) did not want to take medications, I asked her to strongly consider the Pain-Free Diet to see if it might be the answer. And—as I had witnessed with Joseph, Erin, and so many others—within six months, Laurel lost 16 pounds by eating the specific Pain-Free foods outlined in Rx #1, and her back pain was "barely noticeable." In addition, her lab work was now in a normal range.

Substance P and Prostaglandins Send Pain Signals

Other pro-inflammatory markers include *substance P* and *prostaglandins*. Substance P triggers inflammation and pain impulses from the central nervous system. It is thought that when substance P levels are elevated in the body, the person feels more pain. Prostaglandins send messages to cells that trigger inflammation, pain, swelling, and, in some types of arthritis, even joint destruction. In obesity, it is thought there might be a biochemical error that leads to the overproduction of prostaglandins. This gives further support to the importance of weight loss to decrease the resulting inflammation and pain.

You're Only 10 Pounds Away from Reclaiming Control of Your Pain

As your weight continues to escalate over time, you may find yourself suffering with other health problems, including hypertension, abnormal cholesterol levels, or diabetes, along with pain. Your doctor may not be aware that all of these problems are directly associated to your weight and low-grade inflammation in the body. **Stop the cycle!** I want to show you how losing *just 10 pounds*—no matter how much you currently weigh—can decrease concentrations of destructive and painful pro-inflammatory markers. In fact, improving what we call the "inflammatory profile" of fatty tissue in your body may dramatically reduce your pain and risk of other serious illnesses. Most of my patients on this plan report feeling better and more active within just 21 days.

Kate's Low Back Pain

If you met my patient Kate today, you'd have a hard time believing that, just three years ago, she tipped the scales at almost 174 pounds and could barely walk up stairs because of back pain. At age forty-seven, this tall, attractive technical writer was recently divorced and her only son had left home to attend college in another state. Feeling alone, Kate was distressed with all the changes in her life and began to compulsively snack in front of the television for comfort.

Kate initially came to my office because she had no energy, felt much older than she was, and thought she was depressed. She also suffered from low back pain that stemmed from poor posture over the years. When we did initial lab work on Kate, it was obvious that more was going on internally than just anxiety. Her triglycerides and LDL cholesterol were elevated, and her HDL cholesterol was low. Kate's fasting glucose level was also impaired, indicating that her body was in a prediabetic state. And her blood pressure, which she said was normally low-normal, was slightly elevated.

We talked about medications that might be helpful in improving her cholesterol profile, but like so many individuals, Kate was worried about taking medications, and insisted on trying diet and lifestyle changes first. After instituting the four steps in this book, Kate gradually achieved her target weight over a period of eight months. "The unlimited portions of vegetables, fruits, and other foods kept me from feeling hungry," she says.

After the initial 10-pound loss, Kate found it easy to stay on the program as part of a healthy lifestyle. She especially worked on the stress-reduction component (Rx #3). This step helped her to understand why she was eating more than her body needed at night (called stress eating). She also began working out each day at her firm's fitness center, following the specific functional fitness exercises discussed in Rx #2.

Within three weeks of starting the Pain-Free Diet, Kate's lab greatly improved, and by eight months her cholesterol levels were in a healthy range, and her blood pressure and fasting glucose were at normal levels. Kate said her back pain was almost completely resolved, and she only noticed it if she carelessly slumped in her chair while working at the computer or overdid it in her garden on the weekends.

Just a few months after Kate celebrated losing her weight—and the associated inflammation and pain—her son was in an automobile accident and had to have emergency surgery. About the same time, her mother was diagnosed with the early stages of Alzheimer's disease and had to move to a longterm care facility. Normally, either one of these sudden stressful events would have set anyone back in their quest to maintain a normal weight and conquer pain. Nonetheless, Kate held strong to her new lifestyle habits and stuck with the program. Today, she has kept the weight off and continues to enjoy excellent health and manage her pain.

FOUR EASY PRESCRIPTIONS TO END YOUR PAIN

While researchers continue to seek the perfect pill to end pain, I believe there is a better way. Years of clinical research and treating patients have shown that the key intervention to preventing pain is a four-pronged approach that involves the following steps:

Rx I: Eat well and lose weight with the Pain-Free Diet.
Rx 2:   Exercise your pain away.
Rx 3:   Stop the stress-pain connection.
Rx 4:   Increase the quality of your sleep.

Over the past two decades, I have seen repeatedly that the patients who follow this four-step program are the same ones who need less medication, are able to be as active as they want, and experience fewer problems with sleep, anxiety, or fatigue when compared with other overweight or obese patients with pain. To the contrary, my pain patients who are overweight and eat an animal-based diet with few anti-inflammatory foods, who keep erratic hours at night with little sleep and maintain a sedentary, high-stress lifestyle, are the ones who call our clinic frequently, complaining of poor pain control and feelings of achiness, fatigue, insomnia, and depression.

Let's look further at the four prescriptions that make up the Diet for a Pain-Free Life:

Rx #1. Eat Well and Lose Weight with the Pain-Free Diet

"But I hate to diet," you say. "I can't ever seem to stick with one." I reassure you that this is not a deprivation diet! I urge my patients to look at the Pain-Free Diet as a simple way to lose unwanted pounds and decrease pain so they feel great and can be active again. I know that once you begin the diet and take advantage of the variety of foods and recipes for meals and snacks, you will find that you never feel deprived. The pain relief you experience will only reinforce your efforts and help you to stay with the plan.

While there are is no one "magic" food known to cure pain on its own, published studies now associate a reduction in fat storage and pro-inflammatory chemicals in the body with a diet *high* in fresh fruits and vegetables, whole grains, legumes, nuts and seeds, low-fat dairy (including yogurt), and soy products, and *low* in white bread, white rice, and potato products. This mostly plant-based diet also causes an extensive and positive change in the blood fats (triglycerides and LDL and HDL cholesterol) in the body.

Plus, in study after study, researchers have found that key nutrients from the foods recommended in the Pain-Free Diet rival the effects of NSAIDs such as aspirin and ibuprofen, yet without any of the detrimental side effects. If you've lived on NSAIDs for any length of time to ease pain, you've probably experienced the gastrointestinal problems that often occur. With the Pain-Free Diet, you can take advantage of the pain-relieving benefits of anti-inflammatory foods but without the stomach distress of NSAIDs.

Rx #1, Eat Well and Lose Weight with the Pain-Free Diet, offers three different levels that allow you to prepare for weight loss (Level 1: Jump Start), to lose the weight (Level 2: Weight Loss), and then to successfully maintain the weight loss (Level 3: Lifetime). In this section, I explain how the diet works and also give you recipes for the recommended menu plans, so you can select those foods that you enjoy eating.

Initially, you'll be eating around 1,400 calories a day—but, rest assured, you won't feel hungry. The Pain-Free Diet has delicious meals that are high in fiber, which keeps you full as you cut back on calories, saturated and trans fats (both destructive to the body), and potatoes, pasta, and sugary desserts. I'll tell you about changes you can make today in your diet to reduce inflammation, including:

■ Avoiding foods that trigger inflammation such as beef, pork, fried foods, junk food, and grilled food

- Eating anti-inflammatory "good" fats found in olives, fatty fish, and avocados
- Drinking red wine to block inflammation
- Taking anti-inflammatory supplements

To help you successfully conquer pain, in Putting It Into Practice, I outline a 21-day program (page 67) using the recommendations, and also give you scrumptious, quick, and easy "Pain-Free Recipes" (page 111) that use the key anti-inflammatory foods.

Can food choices really make a difference? Yes! My patient Lori lived with severe pain for most of her adult life. In fact, her joint pain was so bad she couldn't even open a jar. Her husband would even unscrew all of the lids in the refrigerator before he left for work.

After seeing a total of ten doctors, Lori came to our clinic and finally received a proper diagnosis—rheumatoid arthritis. Her primary pain trigger? Tomato sauce.

I explained to Lori that some foods seem to increase inflammation in the body, and certain foods decrease it (page 51). For instance, some known arthritis-healing foods include walnuts, olive oil, red grapes, cheese, soy, broccoli, pineapple, and green tea. In addition, a teaspoon of ginger once daily has as much anti-inflammatory effect as some medications.

Changing her diet and adding exercise made all the difference for Lori. She is now 30 pounds lighter and enjoys working out at a nearby fitness center. Lori is in control of her rheumatoid arthritis joint pain instead of letting the pain control her life.

Rx #2. Exercise Your Pain Away

"But I hate to exercise," you say. "I can barely move around as it is!" I know. Most of my patients balk when I explain the importance of exercise to reduce inflammation and pain. Maybe that's because exercise has become complicated, confusing, and even inconvenient. It needn't be. The simple functional fitness exercise regimen in Rx #2 will let you select personalized activities you enjoy, as well as some key stretching movements that can help your joints move in full range of motion and your muscles stay toned. *These exercises have been specifically designed for patients with pain and limited mobility.*

Exercise is a key component of any sound weight-loss regimen. While restricting calories is invariably responsible for the weight loss, regular exercise and activity helps to maintain the weight loss and prevent weight gain. For those with pain, exercise is absolutely essential. Not only does daily exercise and movement help to build stronger muscles to support the joints, it also keeps you flexible, helping you to avoid falls or injury. Exercise also keeps bones strong and helps to prevent fractures, which are painful and debilitating.

My patient Emily detested exercise—as it is defined by most weight-loss books. She said that she owned a treadmill, a stationary bike, and even hand-held dumbbells, but never used any of these to work out. In fact, just looking at her home exercise equipment brought about deep feelings of failure, she said.

In talking with Emily, she mentioned her love for the outdoors and had recently won an award at a county gardening exhibition. I explained to her that exercise does not have to mean walking an hour on a treadmill. Active gardening is superb exercise, and one I always recommend to patients. I find that many people work out longer when they garden because it is enjoyable. You are not restricted to repetitive movement like with a treadmill, and you exercise all joints and muscles. Likewise, window washing, housecleaning, and actively playing with your children or grandchildren are all conditioning exercises as your body moves actively and your heart rate increases. Once Emily began to look at exercise differently, she really got excited about gardening again. Along with her award-winning roses and hibiscus, Emily enjoyed an added benefit—weight loss and less pain.

I've realized through my studies that certain types of exercise boost human growth hormone, which helps in weight reduction and increased muscle tissue. We know that human growth hormone replacement in a person who is deficient results in significant decreases in C-reactive protein, suggesting a decrease in inflammation. It is thought by some that regular exercise, specifically strength training, may give the same result.

In Rx #2, I will show you some easy functional fitness stretches and exercises you can start today to make sure you are doing all you can to build muscle and bone, maintain a normal weight, and, most important, end your pain.

Rx #3. Stop the Stress-Pain Connection

Lillian, age 56, said that just thinking about changing her diet and exercise habits caused her to feel stressed out. Many of my patients claim to have difficulty controlling their daily stress, especially those adults who juggle kids, careers, and other commitments.

Stress is a response of the body to any demand. It is a biological phenomenon that affects the central and autonomic nervous systems, as well as the endocrine and immune systems. The body's major stress hormones trigger the production of pro-inflammatory cytokines, influencing an increased pain response. Stress is linked with changes in our body at a cellular level; changes we don't even feel or see occurring daily until we suddenly experience pain or illness.

Studies show that individuals who are prone to anger, hostility, and depressive symptoms respond to stress with increased production of the stress hormones norepinephrine and cortisol, among others. Scientific evidence suggests that an increase in these stress hormones activates the inflammatory part of the immune system. Remember those pesky C-reactive proteins?

In a fascinating study done at Duke University, healthy volunteers were asked to describe their psychological attributes, including anger, hostility, and depression. The volunteers did not have such conditions as cardiovascular disease or high blood pressure that would predispose them to having high C-reactive protein levels. The researchers used blood tests to measure the C-reactive protein levels and found that the volunteers who were prone to anger and had high hostility levels, and showed mild to moderate symptoms of depression, had two to three times higher C-reactive protein levels than did the calmer volunteers. Researchers concluded that the more pronounced their negative moods, the higher their C-reactive protein levels.

My patient Tavia is an impressive example of someone who suffers from neck pain but who found tremendous improvement after learning to take time out to relax each day. After going through a highly charged divorce, this middle-aged woman was injured in a car accident several years ago. The resulting pain in her neck and shoulders forced her to cut back her work hours to part-time. As a single parent, Tavia depended on her full-time income, so this forced decision greatly increased feelings of anxiety and anger, as well as her stress level and pain.

Tavia met with our clinic psychologist and learned some simple relaxation strategies to deal with her stress and anger, which I will describe here in Rx #3. After practicing these relaxation exercises for three weeks, Tavia said her neck pain was greatly reduced. She was able to resume her fulltime job and for the first time in years, she feels confident that she can deal with life's interruptions in a more positive manner.

There is no "quick fix" for reducing stress or pain. Still, I can help you identify your negative stress response and then learn coping skills to help you respond to life's interruptions in a healthy—not hostile—way.

Rx #4. Increase the Quality of Your Sleep

If you can't sleep, you're not alone—pain is the number-one leading cause of insomnia. Whether from difficulty getting to sleep or problems maintaining sleep, 65 percent of those individuals who suffer from pain claim they "never" get quality sleep. In fact, about 42 million people in the United States report that pain or physical discomfort disrupts their sleep a few nights a week or more. We know that people who have pain experience less deep sleep, more arousals and disruptions with waking, as well as less efficient sleep.

Sleep deprivation (even just an hour a night) results in markedly increased inflammatory cytokines, resulting in pain. Most patients with fibromyalgia, a painful arthritislike syndrome that causes deep muscle aches, fatigue, anxiety, and depression, have difficulty sleeping and feel unrefreshed in the morning. Research shows that many individuals with fibromyalgia have symptoms suggestive of pathologic sleep disturbances like *obstructive sleep apnea (OSA)* (brief periods of cessation of breathing) and restless legs syndrome. In fact, some new studies link pro-inflammatory markers with obstructive sleep apnea. (I'll discuss this fully in Rx #4.)

Sleep disturbances in patients with back, hip, shoulder, neck, or other types of pain can be triggered by the pain itself, by emotional trauma and stress, by a metabolic problem, and by low-grade inflammation. Poor sleep usually leads to feeling fatigued during the day. And this results in a lack of energy for exercise, causing worsened physical fitness and a vicious cycle of inactivity, sleep disturbance, moodiness, and heightened pain sensitivity.

Jordan, a thirty-nine-year-old CPA, was diagnosed with disk disease that caused him tremendous low back pain. For several months before coming to our clinic, Jordan existed on a few hours of sleep each night, as the lower back and hip pain made it difficult for him to get in a comfortable sleep position. After receiving the diagnosis, Jordan began the *Diet for a Pain-Free Life* program. He only needed to lose about 15 pounds, but I felt all of the lifestyle changes would greatly benefit the way Jordan felt each day.

Jordan told me that he slept on a soft mattress that was about twenty years old, and used no pillow under his head. After reading the specific sleep suggestions in this book, he realized that he needed to purchase a new, firm mattress to support his back during sleep. He also added more pillows to his bed so he could sleep on his back with his knees elevated at a right angle (called a 90/90 rest position) on the pillows, helping to take the weight off his hip joints and back. Jordan was astonished that just a few simple changes helped him sleep soundly and awaken with less pain. Not only was he more alert at work, but he was able to get through the day without fatigue and pain.

In Rx #4, I will also elaborate on ways to increase quality sleep to help decrease inflammation, reduce pain, and also to trigger human growth hormone in the body, which can decrease by as much as 75 percent by the time the person is thirty-five years old. Studies show that human growth deficiency leads to obesity, loss of muscle mass, and a reduced capacity to exercise—and getting quality sleep may reverse these problems in older adults.

It's important to note that each of the steps build upon the other to break the pain cycle. For instance, eating the plant-based diet will help you lose weight quickly—without resorting to a strict low-calorie, low carbohydrate or other fad diet. The weight loss will make it easier to move around and exercise more often. Regular exercise helps to boost weight loss and also reduces stress hormones in the body such as cortisol, helping you to feel more relaxed. When you feel relaxed, you are able to fall asleep—and stay asleep throughout the night. Also, for most people, relaxation helps to curb stress eating. Studies also show that each of the four components in this program also decreases inflammation together and independently—and ending inflammation is the key to living pain free.

REAL PATIENTS, REAL RESULTS

Several years ago, I conducted an informal study of 40 of my chronic pain patients who needed to lose weight.* These patients made a firm commitment to follow the four steps in the *Diet for a Pain-Free Life* plan for four months. Before the volunteers began the program, they rated their pain on a scale of 1 to 10 (1 being insignificant pain and 10 being intense pain), using the pain quotient questionnaire on page 26. With this rating system, they were to assign a number to the amount of pain they felt each day and how the pain interfered with their daily activities.

---

* Eleven men and twenty-nine women with the average age of forty-six years.

The volunteer participants did the pain assessment daily for the entire length of the four-month study to see if the four prescriptions—(1) diet and weight loss, (2) daily exercise, (3) stress management, and (4) sleep strategies—actually worked to reduce markers of inflammation and the associated pain.

Upon starting the program, almost all of the volunteers ranked their pain as an 8 or 9 on the 10-point scale. These patients said that pain interfered with most of their daily activities and, while they were able to work and manage a household and family, the volunteers felt that the medications alone were simply not enough to stop the nagging pain and give them a better quality of life.

Prescription #1

For the first month, the volunteers followed the Pain-Free Diet to lose weight. These volunteers reported no problems with compliance to the diet, and all had lost some weight after four weeks (from 2½ pounds to 11 pounds). When the patients assessed their daily pain chart, they noted that the pain was more tolerable after one month on the program. In fact, the average Pain Quotient was now a 6 to 7.

Prescription #2

When the patients started the daily functional fitness exercise program at the beginning of the second month, the feedback was intriguing. First, almost all the patients rated their pain as the same or even slightly higher after seven days of exercise. It's important to note that this was the first time that many of the volunteers had exercised daily in months (or even years), so feeling slightly more pain would be a normal consequence. But as they continued with the diet and exercise regimen, the aches and pains associated with exercise began to subside dramatically. The participants lost more weight and their original pain levels continued to diminish. At the end of 8 weeks of diet and 4 weeks of exercise, only two women rated their pain as higher, and both of these women admitted they had stopped exercising for "fear of more pain." Almost all of the participants rated their pain as a 2 or 3 on the scale.

Prescriptions #3 and #4

As the patients progressed with the Pain-Free program, they continued to lose weight and feel more energetic. At four months, all of the participants reported that their sleep improved as well as their overall response to life's stressors. Not only did their Pain Quotient drop to a group average of 1 to 2 on the pain chart, but the participants claimed their moods also dramatically improved. All of the patients felt positive and hopeful about continuing the program for a lifetime.

WHAT YOU CAN EXPECT FROM THE *DIET FOR A PAIN-FREE LIFE* PROGRAM

- For those who suffer from mild to moderate pain, the four steps in this book will enable you to lose weight, reduce pain, and be more active in as soon as 21 days. Following this program over a period of three months will help you lose 10 to 15 pounds, and to resolve many types of knee, hip, and back pain altogether.
- For those who suffer from moderate to severe pain, this program will complement your doctor's prescribed medications and boost the overall pain-relieving effort, allowing you to lose weight and be more active in just 21 days and notice significantly reduced pain (a drop in 2 to 4 points in your Pain Quotient) over three months as you stay committed to the program.
- For those men and women who suffer from long-term or chronic pain who must turn to surgery or other more invasive procedures, this plan will enable you to lose weight and will help speed recovery and reduce pain.

Medical intervention can sometimes treat daily pain, but it is apparent that our arsenal of protection must target resolving the low-grade inflammation in the body to end the pain altogether. In that regard, suppressing various pro-inflammatory chemicals in the body through the foods you eat and weight loss represents an exciting new therapeutic opportunity for reversing chronic pain.

In the following pages, I'll take you through the four simple steps that have some revolutionary—but quite straightforward—ways to lose weight, feel healthier, and manage your pain. I realize that most people have little time to make healthful dietary choices, so on pages 73 to 143, I have wrapped up the diet prescription for you with a 28-day diet journal with easy-to-follow menu suggestions, as well as food lists and almost thirty recipes. Although I do not know your diet history or lifestyle habits, I do know that if you follow this plan, you can change old behaviors and experience tremendous success in ending the vicious cycle of obesity, inflammation, and pain.

There's no time better than the present to focus on taking care of you. Let's get started!

Rate Your Pain—The Pain Quotient

AS YOU START the Diet for a Pain-Free Life, review these ten questions and then use the following scale to rate your pain each week. By doing so, you can assess how the program is helping to reduce your level of pain and whether you need to check with your doctor for a change in medication if your pain level stays the same or even increases. I will refer to this scale throughout the book, so be sure to photocopy this page and keep a weekly chart of your Pain Quotient (score).

0 = no pain   10 = worst pain imaginable

0   1   2   3   4   5   6   7   8   9   10

Now circle a number that reflects how the pain you feel interferes with each of the following areas:

0 = no interference   10 = total interference

1. Ability to walk

0   1   2   3   4   5   6   7   8   9   10

2. Ability to perform activities of daily living (household chores, dressing)

0   1   2   3   4   5   6   7   8   9   10

3. Mood

0   1   2   3   4   5   6   7   8   9   10

4. Sleep

0   1   2   3   4   5   6   7   8   9   10

5. Enjoyment of life

0   1   2   3   4   5   6   7   8   9   10

6. Relationship with significant other(s)

0   1   2   3   4   5   6   7   8   9   10

7. Recreational activities

0   1   2   3   4   5   6   7   8   9   10

8. Sexual activities

0   1   2   3   4   5   6   7   8   9   10

9. Amount of social interaction

0   1   2   3   4   5   6   7   8   9   10

10. Productivity at home and in the workplace

0   1   2   3   4   5   6   7   8   9   10

Calculate Your Pain Score

Now add together all the numbers you circled and divide by ten. The resulting number is your *Pain Quotient*. Keep track of your Pain Quotient each week. As you follow the four steps in the Pain-Free Diet, you should notice a continual decline in your Pain Quotient, which is an indicator that you are showing improvement and starting to enjoy the benefits of weight loss, reduced inflammation, and decreased pain. (Many of my patients report a 2- to 3-point decrease in their Pain Quotient after just 21 days on the program.) But if your pain increases at any time while you are following the 4-step program, and/or taking prescribed medications, talk to your doctor for an evaluation. You might need a change of medication, or there may be another reason for the pain.

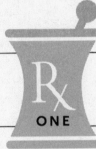

ONE

Eat Well and Lose Weight with the Pain-Free Diet

Eat Well and Lose Weight with the Pain-Free Diet

The easiest, least expensive way to end pain is to lose weight.

SINCE I STARTED my internal medicine practice in 1978, I have watched some of the most vital men and women become inactive and even dependent on caregivers as they moved into middle age and began to live with the results of having ignored their weight. Not only did their excess poundage greatly burden their muscles, joints, and bones, but it also caused a painful, pro-inflammatory state in the body, impacting their health and ability to be active. Many of these patients had been athletes in high school and college. Others thrived on busy weekends, engaging in recreational and competitive sports or active gardening. Yet, in an almost predictable way, as these overweight baby-boomer men and women hit forty and beyond, they would come to my office with a host of health problems such as hypertension, diabetes, and cardiovascular disease, along with joint and muscle pain and stiffness.

You might think it odd that a *rheumatologist* who specializes in *arthritis* and related diseases has written a weight-loss program. But the reasoning is quite sound—many of these problems follow an established pattern and are often the result of obesity, which triggers a powerful pro-inflammatory state in the body. This biochemical state is partially the result of a calorie-laden diet filled with too much meat and fried or sugar-laden, overprocessed foods—fried chicken, pizza, fast-food burgers and fries, and rich desserts—and not enough fruits, vegetables, and whole grains. I determined early on in my medical practice to find realistic nutritional solutions for my patients to help them lose weight to reduce and manage their pain. The Pain-Free Diet described in this key step is that solution.

The Pain-Free Diet (plant based, with eggs, low-fat dairy, fish, and occasionally poultry) is a moderately low-carbohydrate (MLC) plan that regulates calories, fats, protein, and carbohydrates. Because it is higher in protein and healthy monounsaturated fats than most weight-loss diets, it helps to curb hunger pangs and allows you to enjoy a host of complex carbohydrates, while still losing weight. It has been shown in clinical trials that an MLC plan is more effective in reducing blood lipids and markers of inflammation, as well as your weight, than is a low-fat, high-carbohydrate diet. With the Pain-Free Diet, you will eliminate most animal foods from the diet and increase *anti-inflammatory* plant foods to significantly reduce weight and low-grade inflammation—and thus reduce chronic pain.

In this chapter, I will explain to you why the Pain-Free Diet is the most proven and effective eating style for losing weight and decreasing inflammation at the same time. I'll give you the details on some anti-inflammatory nutrients found in foods and how they work together to stop pain. I also have lists of specific foods you can snack on while on this diet, so you feel full and energetic while your body is dropping pounds. Lastly, although I'm a strong proponent of eating whole foods to get all the available nutrients for the body, I recommend some Pain-Free natural dietary supplements you might consider taking. There is increasing scientific evidence that these supplements can help to boost optimal health, decrease markers of inflammation, and ease pain.

Julie's Hypertension and Prediabetes

Last year, I diagnosed Julie with hypertension (high blood pressure) and prediabetes at the early age of forty-two. This exuberant mother of three works in computer software sales and spends most of her day sitting—either in her office while setting up appointments or in her car as she drives to meet with clients. A few years before I first saw Julie, she had been injured in an automobile accident and since had suffered with tremendous back and neck pain. The pain, which she rated a level 8 to 9, caused her to shy away from exercise; since the accident, Julie said, she had gained about 20 pounds.

When Julie heard the diagnosis, she knew she had to get in control of her lifestyle and eating habits. The alternative of taking medications for the rest of her life was just not acceptable to her. I shared that some new studies among perimenopausal overweight women, like Julie, found that losing just 10 pounds is associated with a significant reduction in inflammatory markers, reduced pain, and even reversal of problems like high blood pressure and diabetes.

I convinced Julie to switch to the Pain-Free Diet. Admittedly, at first she laughed, wondering how she could ever convince her teenage sons and husband to eat stir-fried broccoli with red peppers and pecan-crusted salmon for dinner, when they thrived on pepperoni pizza and greasy Chinese food. But when Julie saw that I was not laughing, she committed to changing her dietary habits in order to get well—and did.

WHY A PLANT-BASED DIET? WHY NOW?

Many of my patients initially respond as Julie did when I first recommend a plant-based diet filled with powerful anti-inflammatory compounds. But I hope you will listen and take the information to heart. As an internist and pain specialist, I am convinced that a predominantly plant-based diet is what it will take for millions of Americans to get off the epidemic obesity bandwagon and finally lose extra weight in order to have a pain-free, active lifestyle. Especially with 2 out of 3 adult Americans overweight or clinically obese, it's time we all took this problem very seriously and made a commitment to long-term solutions that are quick, safe, and effective (and still taste good).

Over the past decade, there have been a multitude of scientific studies supporting a plant-based eating style for both weight loss and optimal health. Some recent findings reveal that a plant-based diet not only increases weight loss, but it actually prevents certain diseases, by targeting pro-inflammatory markers that silently increase over time.

In a study published in the journal *Nutrition Reviews*, researchers compiled data from eighty-seven previous diet studies and concluded that, while obesity is skyrocketing in the general population in the United States, it only affects about *0 to 6 percent of vegetarians*. Vegetarians also have a much lower rate of heart disease, diabetes, hypertension, and other serious conditions that are often linked to excess body fat.

While losing weight or being a normal weight is necessary to avoid such problems as hypertension and diabetes with aging, we are just now beginning to learn how a plant-based diet can decrease the markers of inflammation in the body—inflammation that increases the pain you feel.

Super-antioxidants Reduce Inflammation

Substantial evidence implicates *oxygen free radicals* as agents of inflammation and tissue destruction in many types of pain disorders. Free radicals are the unstable by-products of oxidation, the chemical process that causes iron to rust and a peeled apple or banana to turn brown. In the body, free radicals cause similar deterioration, as they destroy cell membranes and make cells vulnerable to decay and pathogens. These free radicals damage DNA and mitochondria, the basic building blocks of all tissues, and leave in their path many health problems.

We cannot stop free radicals completely. Yet we can reduce their pro-inflammatory effect on the body by eating foods high in powerful *antioxidants*— plant chemicals that scavenge and neutralize the free radicals. So far, the known antioxidants include vitamin C, vitamin E, selenium, the carotenoids, which have immune-boosting properties, and the flavonoids, plant compounds that reportedly have antiviral, anti-inflammatory, and antitumor activities. Recently, there has been a deluge of scientific studies revealing that many compounds found in fruits, vegetables, and even whole grains also have antioxidant properties— some more potent than others.

As an example, in laboratory findings published last year, researchers found that "purple berries" are as much as 50 percent higher in antioxidants than some of the more common antioxidant-rich fruits. In another recent study by the USDA, researchers analyzed antioxidant levels of more than one hundred different foods. They concluded that cranberries, blueberries, and blackberries ranked highest in antioxidants among the fruits studied; artichokes, beans, and russet potatoes had the highest of all the vegetables; and hazelnuts, walnuts, and pecans had the highest antioxidants levels in the nut category.

Many nutrition researchers who test the antioxidant activity of foods believe that certain foods reduce the risk of some degenerative diseases associated with aging, such as arthritis, heart disease, diabetes, and cancer. But findings on arthritis patients published in the journal *Nutrition and Metabolism* concluded that those individuals who adopted a plant-based diet high in *super-antioxidants* also obtained a reduction in pain and disease activity, and an improvement in physical function and vitality. These changes are thought to favor the production of anti-inflammatory chemicals in the body. Anti-inflammatory chemicals actually target and eliminate the pro-inflammatory markers. The many different foods in the Pain-Free Diet have other anti-inflammatory nutrients besides super-antioxidants.

While the results from these scientific studies are impressive to read, I believe we must take these studies to the next level in an effort to implement these findings in our diet. So I have asked my daughter, Virginia McIlwain, a graduate of Le Cordon Bleu Culinary Academy, if she could use these super-antioxidants, along with other anti-inflammatory foods, to create scrumptious but low-calorie dishes. Virginia has an impressive résumé, having studied with preeminent chefs in the United States and abroad, and completing her externship at the L'Ecrivain, an award-winning restaurant in Dublin, Ireland. She spent months researching the super-antioxidants and other foods used in the Pain-Free Diet, and then created the superb menu choices, beginning on page 71.

Top 20 Pain-Free Super-Antioxidants*

1. Small red beans
2. Wild blueberries
3. Red kidney beans
4. Pinto beans
5. Cultivated blueberries
6. Cranberries
7. Artichokes
8. Blackberries
9. Prunes
10. Raspberries
11. Strawberries
12. Red delicious/granny smith apples
13. Pecans
14. Sweet cherries
15. Black plums
16. Russet potatoes
17. Black beans
18. Plums
19. Gala apples
20. Walnuts

* As established by the United States Department of Agriculture

Go Ahead! Feel Full and Weigh Less

For years I have enjoyed talking openly with patients about their eating habits and listening carefully to their responses. Invariably, those patients who eat a plant-based diet and who are at or near a normal weight are usually the ones who have had less disease, better pain control, healthier lab results, and more active lives.

Not only are plant-based diets proven to be healthier, they have high water content yet are low in calories. This allows you to feel full before you are tempted to add another serving to your plate. In fact, numerous studies show that vegetarians weigh significantly less than nonvegetarians as measured by body mass index (BMI) or body weight. I concur with those experts who believe that the vegetarian's lower average body weight is linked to the high fiber content of the plant foods. Plant fiber fills you up quickly, and studies indicate that this results in less snacking and bingeing later in the day. But a high-fiber diet has another key benefit that is scientifically proven: it protects against high levels of C-reactive protein and other inflammatory markers in the body.

Calories Do Count!

NO MATTER WHAT the popular fad diets claim, calories count. *You cannot lose weight without burning more calories than you consume each day.* The American Dietetic Association (ADA) recommends a calorie level of no less than ten times your desired weight, with women getting at least 1,200 calories and men getting at least 1,400 per day. For example, if your goal is to be 140 pounds, you should eat around 1,400 calories per day. The target daily calorie count in the Pain-Free Diet is 1,400 calories. However, if your goal is 170 pounds, you might need to add more calories, up to 1,700 calories each day. While you might not see a rapid reduction of weight following this rule, the chances of *keeping the weight off* are much greater. And as you stay on the diet and increase daily exercise, you will lose weight even faster.

THE THREE LEVELS

Let's be honest: losing weight is not easy. The older you get, the more difficult it is to drop pounds. On many of today's fad diets, even if you do lose weight, the chance of gaining it all back is huge. That's why I recommend that my patients adopt this medically proven diet, which is plant based, plus fish, low-fat dairy, and eggs. A quasi-vegetarian diet will let you eat *more* food and have *even* larger portions than a nonvegetarian diet, while consuming *fewer* calories. Aside from that, the recommended foods are filled with potent *phytochemicals*, the biologically active substances that give plants their deep colors, flavors, odors, and protection against disease.

To help you stay on the diet and lose weight at a steady pace, I have divided the Pain-Free Diet into three distinct levels:

LEVEL 1: Jump Start
LEVEL 2: Weight Loss
LEVEL 3: Lifetime

LEVEL 1: Jump Start

This level of the diet is portion and calorie controlled, and offers plant-based foods (fruits, vegetables, and some whole grains), along with fish and eggs (egg whites and egg substitutes). You will be on this level for fourteen days.

During the **Jump Start,** you will detoxify your body of years of unhealthy eating. You will eat about 1,400 calories per day, but the meals are designed to be filling. This particular level is moderately lower in carbohydrates and higher in good fats and protein than most diets. This combination gives the added benefit of curbing your appetite, so you won't feel like snacking in the late afternoon or bingeing at night while watching television. In clinical trials, a moderately low-carbohydrate diet has been found to be more effective in reducing excess weight and the levels of inflammatory markers in the body than the low-fat, high carbohydrate diet or the low-carb, high protein (meat eater) diet.

The Upside: You can have delicious high-fiber fruits, vegetables, soy products (even popular brands), fish, and eggs, among some whole-grain products and other foods. You can also enjoy "free" snack foods (page 109) that are easy to take with you to work, the tennis court, or while carpooling kids to after-school activities.

The Downside: You may not have alcohol (Two weeks is *not* forever!). You will also cut out white sugar, white flour, white potatoes, pasta, and whole dairy products. The only "white" foods you can eat during the first two weeks are fish, egg whites, white beans, tofu, and low-fat dairy products.

The Bonus: You should feel extremely satisfied the first two weeks, and will lose from 2 to 7 pounds or more by the end of this period if you follow the diet plan carefully—and are cautious with your portion sizes. Your pain level may also drop 2 to 4 points—which will be incentive for you to continue this diet and lifestyle plan.

LEVEL 2: Weight Loss

This second level is portion and calorie controlled (1,400) and also plant based (fruits, vegetables, and whole grains), plus fish and eggs. With **Weight Loss**, you will add low-fat dairy products, red wine, and dessert. **Weight Loss** is higher in protein and complex carbohydrates and lower in fat than **Jump Start**, but you will still feel full, making it easy to stay compliant to the plan. You will stay on this level until you reach or are close to your desired weight—perhaps weeks, perhaps months, depending on how many pounds you need to lose and how successfully you maintain this regimen.

Level 2 offers greater varieties of food, incredible recipes created specifically for this diet, and more freedom in selecting your menu options. I want you to stay on **Weight Loss** until you have lost most of your weight (or are within 5 to 10 pounds of your goal weight). For some people, this might be one to four months; for others, it can be nine months to a year or longer.

No matter how long it takes to lose the weight, I *never* want you to feel deprived. And if you do feel deprived, please take several bites of the food you are craving and restart the diet at the next meal.

The Pain-Free Diet is meant to be one you can stay with for life—so you can be pain-free for life. It is not effective if you use it for 3 weeks and then resume eating the way you used to. If you begin to regularly add back foods such as beef, high-calorie snack foods, and baked goods, I can almost guarantee you that your pain will return, along with increased levels of pro-inflammatory markers in your body.

Unlike a typical low-carbohydrate diet like Atkins, which allows bacon, steak, butter, and cream, **Weight Loss** allows generous portions of vegetables, fruits, legumes, fish, low-fat dairy, eggs, and whole grains. We now know that people who eat foods high in saturated fats—most often found in animal products such as bacon, steak, butter, and cream, pay the price with more *prostaglandins*, which are chemicals in the body that cause inflammation, pain, swelling, and in some types of arthritis, even joint destruction. It's the pain caused by prostaglandins that bothers most of us.

Because of the unique variety of food offerings (see page 111), **Weight Loss** is basically lower in calories but much higher in food volume than most popular diets, and lets you feel full while losing weight faster. A quasi-vegetarian diet such as this makes your body more responsive to insulin, offering a great benefit to those who already have signs of metabolic syndrome or prediabetes. And because the body is more responsive to insulin, you don't get powerful hunger pangs, making it easier to stay with the diet. As you drop pounds, the levels of pro-inflammatory markers in the body decrease, reducing or even ending the pain you feel. This in itself is great reinforcement to continue following the Pain-Free Diet!

> **The Upside:** You can have delicious fruits, vegetables, whole grains, prepared soy products, nuts and seeds, fish, eggs, and low-fat dairy, among other foods. You may also have a glass of red wine daily.
>
> **The Downside:** There are not too many negatives about **Weight Loss**, although you may feel cravings. If you crave a hamburger, you should try to refrain (for now). If you must have meat to satisfy a craving, chicken or turkey are better choices. Remind yourself of your goal of losing weight and ending your pain.
>
> **The Bonus:** You can have a favorite dessert or rich snack (250 to 300 calories) once per week.

LEVEL 3: Lifetime

This level starts when you are at or near your goal weight. **Lifetime** is portion controlled and plant based, plus fish, eggs, low-fat dairy, and even poultry, if desired. You add calories at this point, if you can do so without gaining weight. As the title of this level suggests, this is the plan you should continue to use to maintain your ideal weight. Just be sure to drop back to **Weight Loss** if you find yourself gaining weight again.

Again, after you've dropped the first 10 pounds and moved closer to your weight-loss goal, add poultry (chicken or turkey without skin) if you'd like. While most of my patients truly enjoy the quasi-vegetarian style of eating, other patients cannot undertake a diet plan without meat—they enjoy poultry and must have it to be compliant to the diet. If you must have some type of meat, eat poultry at any time on this diet. Don't let that be a stumbling block.

The Upside: On **Lifetime,** you continue to eat fruits, unlimited nonstarchy vegetables, whole grains, soy products, nuts and seeds, fish, eggs and egg substitutes, and low-fat dairy, among other foods. You still drink the glass of red wine each day.

The Downside: There is no downside! You are near your weight goal; you look and feel great!

The Bonus: Continue to have a favorite dessert or snack (250 to 300 calories) once per week. When you reach your goal weight, you can increase this to twice weekly if you can maintain your goal weight.

So, Where's the Beef?

Not surprisingly, there is *no* beef . . . or pork or lamb on the Pain-Free Diet. You will not eat bacon, ham, steak, duck, pork loin, veal chops, or any of the other high-saturated-fat animal foods that are offered on popular low-carb diets. You will not snack on lunch meat, cocktail sausages, pepperoni, or hot dogs, either. Aside from this, you can add poultry (chicken or turkey) to your diet if you'd like, but I'd like you to wait until you've dropped the first 10 pounds.

The plant-based Pain-Free Diet is completely different from the South Beach, Zone, Atkins, Perricone Weight-Loss, and other popular diets today that promote eating meat (a scientifically proven *pro-inflammatory* food). Some important journal studies confirm that meat contains high amounts of *arachidonic acid.* This fatty acid is converted to pro-inflammatory chemicals that lead to disease, inflammation, and increased pain. If you want to decrease inflammation and live pain free, you *simply must forgo the meat* (particularly beef, pork, and lamb) and learn to focus instead on healing, plant-based foods and fish that offer true benefit to your body.

Dessert and Wine Are Served

So many of my patients thrive on this diet because it allows them to have a glass of red wine each day and a rich dessert once a week (and more often, after they have lost most of their weight). I recommend fruit desserts to take advantage of the super-antioxidants and other healing plant nutrients in berries, apples, and melons. But I will admit, chocolate is my favorite dessert. Interestingly, chocolate is filled with healing antioxidants and flavonoids, and compares to kale, spinach, and brussels sprouts when it comes to absorbing oxygen free radicals. If you love chocolate, I hope you will select this for your weekly splurge!

The Pain-Free Diet and Meat

MY PATIENT ROB, age 43, needed to start the Pain-Free Diet to lose weight and also to end the constant knee pain he had battled since playing college basketball at the University of Florida. But when our practice's dietitian explained the variety of foods to him, he balked: Rob had to have meat!

We encouraged Rob to continue eating poultry, particularly skinless chicken or turkey—and to carefully watch his portion sizes and try to diversify his meals with the other protein substitutes. Rob made the commitment to the Pain-Free Diet, lost 35 pounds over a period of six months, and was able to cut back to only one anti-inflammatory medication, taken only as needed. He also took up long-distance cycling with some co-workers, and now spends his weekends competing in bicycling marathons in the United States and abroad. While the cycling helps to burn calories, allowing Rob to eat more calories and maintain his new weight, this exercise also strengthens the important muscles that support his injured knee—a double benefit.

CREATING THE SQUARE MEAL

Most people have heard the term *square meal*. In years past, a *square meal* referred to having a substantial, nourishing meal. When I first designed the Pain-Free Diet, I realized that my patients would need a very specific—and easy—way to monitor their portion sizes. Thus, I started using the term *Square Meal* to describe the structure of the meals.

I have found that by planning meals following this structure, you can eat almost anywhere—at home, work, and restaurants—and stay within a safe calorie range. You can also eat the balanced ratio of complex carbohydrates, good fats, and plant-based protein (or eggs, fish and low-fat dairy) to satisfy your appetite, lose weight, and reduce inflammation and pain.

In creating your own Square Meal, I want you to envision a square on your regular plate. Now divide the square into four equal sections, filling in each section as follows:

1. **One-fourth** of the square will be filled with the recommended protein.
   - The serving of recommended protein will have from 100 to 150 calories at lunch; 150 to 200 calories at dinner.
   - The serving will include soy and soy-based products, legumes (beans, peas, and lentils), eggs, fish, nuts and seeds, and poultry, if desired. Protein lists are on pages 105 to 106.
2. **One-fourth** of the square will be filled with high-protein pasta; brown rice; whole-grain pasta; or high-fiber, whole-grain bread, chosen from the list on page 105.
   - The serving of recommended whole grains will have about 75 calories at lunch; 150 calories at dinner. If you use the Pain-Free Diet recipes, this section of your plate may be used for the particular recipe, if stated.
3. **One-fourth** of the square will have unlimited low-starch vegetables, chosen from the abundant list on page 104.
   - One serving of low-starch vegetables will have from 15 to 30 calories. Please feel free to have seconds or even thirds!
4. **One-fourth** of the square will have super-antioxidant fruits, such as berries, apples, red grapes, pomegranate, and pineapple, chosen from the list on page 103.
   - One serving of the super-antioxidant fruits will have from 25 to 50 calories.

What about Breakfast?

On the Pain-Free Diet, your breakfast may not literally be in quarters on a plate, but will pretty much follow the same pattern—that is, a very high-protein egg-white omelet with roasted vegetables and low-fat cheese or berries, nonfat or low-fat yogurt with fruit and nuts, or a bowl of hot oatmeal with fresh berries, among other delicious suggested selections (pages 120 to 125).

A Sample Daily Menu

The total calorie count of the breakfast with the two Square Meals is about 1,100 calories daily. I also want you to add one low-fat dairy item (skim milk or yogurt) or calcium-fortified soy milk to your daily meal plan. You can have the milk or yogurt with your meal—or use this for one of your snacks or in your hot coffee or tea. You will also get skim milk or calcium-fortified soy milk in your daily Berry Nice Smoothie (page 113). I recommend taking a calcium supplement, as described on page 63.

Aside from all these choices, you will add two low-calorie snacks (choosing from the list on pages 108 to 109) for a total of 1,250 calories. You can then add a 5-ounce glass of red wine, rich in anti-inflammatory compounds, when you reach the Weight Loss and Lifetime levels.

As you become accustomed to dividing your plate into four sections categorized as protein, whole grains, nonstarchy vegetables, and fruits, be really creative and select the foods that you enjoy eating—but also those that will boost weight loss and decrease inflammation. For example, during Weight Loss, your Pain-Free Diet menu for the day might look something like the following. (I noted the calories of each food in parenthesis, so you can see how the total day adds up.)

BREAKFAST

½ cup Eggbeaters (Cheese and Chive) (70)

½ Thomas' Hearty Grain Muffin with 2 teaspoons low-sugar fruit jelly (90)

Hot green tea (0)

SNACK:

1 cup Dr. McIlwain's Anytime Vegetable Soup (0)

LUNCH

1 whole-grain pita (150)

¼ cup water-packed albacore tuna with 2 teaspoons light mayo (70) mixed with ½ cup white cannellini beans and ½ teaspoon Italian seasoning (100)

8 ripe green olives, sliced (40), added to salad

Chopped romaine lettuce, green onion, red pepper strips (stuff the salad into pita bread)

½ cup halved strawberries (25)

SNACK

1 medium-size apple, sliced (57)

2 teaspoons peanut butter (95), for dipping apple

DINNER

4 ounces grouper with lemon, salt, and pepper (130), broiled with olive oil cooking spray

1½ cups fresh green beans (60)

½ cup brown rice with scallions (100)

2 slices fresh pineapple (20)

5 ounces red wine

EVENING SNACK

½ cup nonfat yogurt with ½ cup strawberries (75)

SAMPLE DAY'S ANTI-INFLAMMATORY FOODS:

Albacore tuna

Apple

Green olives

Grouper

Peanut butter

Pineapple

Red wine

Salad: shredded romaine lettuce, green onion, red pepper strips

Strawberries

White cannellini beans (white kidney beans)

Total Calories with red wine: 1,350

If you plan your meals ahead of time, they can be filled with very satisfying anti-inflammatory foods such as those in the sample meal plan (see page 71) and also stay within the calorie limit necessary for you to lose weight (1,400 average). As you drop pounds, the pro-inflammatory markers in your body will also decrease. You will become thinner and have more energy, but, most important, you will see a remarkable difference in your pain threshold and overall health.

On pages 71 to 111, I will help you get started in planning your meals by giving you sample daily food choices, along with specific instructions for all three Pain-Free Diet levels. Also in this section, delicious recipes with serving sizes and nutritional information for the recommended menus are given for each level.

Downsizing Portions

Portion control is a touchy subject for many people, especially for those who enjoy the way most restaurants today supersize meals. After all, with some of the popular fad diets, you are allowed *unlimited* amounts of high-calorie, low-carb foods. But how do we monitor unlimited amounts knowing we all have different appetites and rates of metabolism? Appetite regulation is a very complicated mechanism, and it seems likely that we all respond differently.

You must assess portion sizes with any diet. We know that large portions—the "supersize" factor—play a central role in the current obesity epidemic in America. A recent series of studies showed how easily people fall into the habit of consuming oversized portions. In one trial, researchers tracked the food consumption of nearly two dozen adults for 11 days. First, they gave the volunteers twelve standard-size servings, followed by portions that were 50 percent larger. The participants consistently ate more when they were given more to eat. The only limit the participants in this study placed on themselves was for vegetables—they didn't eat as many of them as they did of the other types of food available. I read recently that the average American adult eats only 1½ servings of fruits and vegetables each day. Is it any wonder that obesity and chronic pain are at epidemic proportions?

How Much Is a Serving?

THE AMERICAN DIABETES Association recommends the following analogy as a way of measuring one serving of a certain food:

- A ½-cup serving of canned fruit, vegetables, or potatoes looks like half a tennis ball.
- Three ounces of meat, fish, or chicken is about the size of a deck of playing cards or the palm of your hand.
- A 1-ounce serving of cheese is about the size of your thumb.
- A 1-cup serving of milk, yogurt, or fresh greens is about the size of your fist.
- One teaspoon of oil is about the size of your thumb tip.

As you follow the Pain-Free Diet, I urge you to stay with the recommended serving size as detailed in my description of the Square Meal, and as described below by the American Diabetes Association. If you cheat by miscalculating your serving sizes, the only person you are cheating is yourself. If your portions are accurate, it is quite likely you will meet your weight-loss and pain-management goals.

Lynn's 2,400-Calorie Weight-Loss Diet

IT'S TYPICAL FOR us to underestimate how much we're really eating. In the beginning, it can be helpful to keep a food and portion diary to ensure you're staying on track. Lynn, a forty-nine-year-old preschool teacher, suffered with neck and shoulder pain and initially needed to lose about 15 pounds to see her goal weight of 140. At each office visit, she assured me that she was following the Pain-Free Diet. Yet Lynn continued to gain weight between visits until her weight topped at 160 pounds. I finally asked Lynn to record her daily food intake.

After three weeks, Lynn brought in a record of what she had been eating. Instead of staying around 1,400 calories, which she "estimated," Lynn was averaging around 2,200 to 2,400 calories daily—almost a thousand calories more than her small-framed, five-foot-two body could use for weight loss. After reviewing her food diary and showing her the real calorie calculations, Lynn saw "in writing" where she had overindulged. She promised to carefully keep track of the foods and portions she ate, and to continue her daily exercise program.

When Lynn returned again in three months, she had lost 15 pounds and had dramatically changed her eating habits. The benefits of a slimmer waistline, more energy, and a reduction in neck and shoulder pain gave Lynn the motivation needed to stick with the plan.

What You Can Expect

After following the 2-week Jump Start on the Pain-Free Diet, you should lose approximately 2 to 7 pounds or even more, depending on your size and compliance to the program. Once you have dropped 10 pounds on Weight Loss, which can take from 4 to 16 weeks, add chicken or turkey to your diet, if you enjoy eating meat. If you enjoy the predominantly plant-based diet, I urge you to continue with this anti-inflammatory eating style to increase weight loss and decrease inflammation and pain. Over the long term, the quasi-vegetarian diet will help you maintain your weight loss goals and feel tremendous relief from pain.

Frank's Incredible Results after Just 6 Days

FRANK, AGE 66, contacted me through e-mail inquiring about the Pain-Free Diet. Frank said he suffered with obstructive sleep apnea, type 2 diabetes, and osteoarthritis of the knee, and needed a diet for life that would help him lose weight and decrease inflammation. (Obesity and inflammation are both related to obstructive sleep apnea, diabetes, and osteoarthritis.)

Frank wrote, "I am only 5 foot 6 inches and weigh about 325 lbs. My waist is about 59–60 inches and I haven't measured my hips in a long time. Recently, I have had problems getting out of my chair because of low back and hip pain and even short walks to get the mail result in tremendous pain and stiffness. I lost 95 lbs. on an old Weight Watchers program and kept it off for two years. Then, I put it all back on again. I tried the Cybervision diet and lost just over 50 lbs., then switched to Physicians' Weight Loss. That one put me in ketosis intentionally. I lost 127 lbs. on that one and got down to 174 lbs., but my skin was gray in color and my liver enzymes were elevated. Since then, I have tried Richard Simmons's Deal-a-Meal, the Atkins diet, and then the South Beach diet. I have even taken a scale to restaurants. I have counted calories, carbs, and points. Needless to say, I must have a very fuel-efficient metabolism. At 66, losing weight will probably be a lot more difficult, but I sure would like to give it an honest try."

Frank followed the instructions on page 110 for removing pro-inflammatory foods from his pantry and refrigerator.

After just six days on the Pain-Free Diet, Frank wrote, "Today I saw my primary care physician. He was pleased that I had started this diet, and the fact that I have lost 8½ pounds in less than a week was good. However, even better was the fact that I have been almost entirely pain-free today without using any pain medication at all. I feel good about what I am doing and have more energy than I have had in a long time."

SELECTING PAIN-FREE FOODS

Now that you have a better understanding of the three levels of the Pain–Free Diet, the Square Meal servings, and how portion size can make or break your weight-loss goals, I want to tell you about the anti-inflammatory foods. These foods have been carefully selected for a specific purpose or function, and that is to help you to lose weight quickly, decrease pro-inflammatory markers in your body, and reduce or end pain altogether. There is some scientific evidence that these Pain-Free foods give an added bonus of an increased "calorie burn" after meals, as the foods are used efficiently as fuel for the body instead of being stored as fat.

Eliminate These Foods Starting Today

THERE ARE SEVERAL key ways inflammation is triggered in the body. For instance, eating too much saturated fat causes an increase in C-reactive protein—a pro-inflammatory marker (see page 7). Eating starchy foods such as white potatoes, white breads, and pastries promotes excess production of IL-6 (discussed on page 13). To gain optimal benefit from the Pain-Free Diet, be sure to *eliminate or at least eat less of the following foods*:

- *Animal protein such as red meat, butter, and whole milk* because they contain arachidonic acid, a fatty acid that is converted to pro-inflammatory chemicals in the body that trigger pain.

- *Foods cooked at high temperatures*, including snack foods, french fries, packaged crackers, and chips. Fried foods are also high in the unhealthy trans fats, which come from adding hydrogen to vegetable oil through a process called hydrogenation. You can check the package's nutritional facts to see if a food has trans fats. Because of the greater awareness of the danger of trans fats, some manufacturers put "trans fat free" on packages of foods that do not contain these unhealthy fats; however, be aware that these foods may still contain high levels of sugar, salt, or processed starches.

- *Snack foods that contain sugar and processed starches.* The inflammatory process is triggered by surges of insulin, which increases the risk of obesity and pro-inflammatory chemicals in the body. Studies show excessive consumption of sugars and starchy carbohydrates (white bread, white flour, potatoes) can trigger spikes of insulin in the body, worsening inflammation in the body. Always review the nutrition facts on a product to check for added sugars. You can also read the ingredients and check for such terms as *corn syrup* and *high fructose corn syrup*, which indicate added sugar. Remember that honey, molasses, and glucose, dextrose, and fructose are all sugars.

- *Foods that trigger allergic reactions* (if you have problems with these foods), which may include corn, eggs, beef, seafood, yeast, soy, and dairy products. Aside from making you feel bad from the reaction itself, subjecting your body to these foods places extra stress upon your immune system. Your goal is to eliminate stress.
- *Nightshade plants* such as potatoes, tomatoes, peppers, and eggplant, which are thought to worsen inflammation, if these foods bother you. Although nightshade plants don't bother most individuals with pain, some of my patients are sensitive to the chemical alkaloid called solanine, which can trigger inflammation and pain. If you believe these foods do not affect your inflammation or pain, you can continue to eat them.

---

5 Ways Pain-Free Foods Provide Optimal Healing

1. **Phytochemicals stop inflammation.** The bulk of the Pain-Free Diet is based on high fiber and colorful fruits and vegetables and whole grains that are filled with *phytochemicals* (also called phytonutrients). These chemicals or nutrients derived from plants provide a beneficial effect on health, as well as play an active role in resolving disease. Not only are these foods filled with fiber that helps to prevent diseases such as type 2 diabetes, but fruits, vegetables, and whole grains taste good, fill you up, and are loaded with anti-inflammatory compounds.

2. **Vitamin C builds cartilage.** A study published in the *American Journal of Clinical Nutrition* reported that high blood levels of vitamin C were associated with a 45 percent reduced risk of inflammation, and high fruit intake was related to a 25 percent reduced risk of inflammation. As an antioxidant, vitamin C also protects DNA from free radical damage, which helps to control inflammation in the body, and plays a part in rebuilding and regenerating damaged joint tissue.

   But there are other healing benefits from fruits and vegetables that are not directly related to inflammation. Scientists have long noted that vitamin C plays a key role in building and protecting collagen. Collagen is an important part of the cartilage, which cushions the joints as they move. In osteoarthritis, the cartilage wears away and becomes less efficient. Seeking ways to offset the fact that your ability to maintain normal cartilage structure decreases with age, some comprehensive studies show that specific compounds in cherries, blackberries, and blueberries help in cartilage formation and prevent cartilage destruction. Less cartilage destruction means less pain and greater mobility as you age. As an added benefit, berries (particularly raspberries) also contain ellagic acid, a chemical that might help fight cancer.

3. **Berries contain super-antioxidants.** Likewise, grapes, mulberries, and bilberries contain pterostilbene, a natural antioxidant with anti-inflammatory, antioxidant, and immunomodulatory activities. This super-antioxidant lowers blood glucose and may be a potent antidiabetic agent. In addition, garlic, onions, and cabbage increase the sulfur content of the body. Sulfur is necessary for the formation of connective tissue and plays a role in the production of collagen.

4. **Flavonoids boost immunity.** Flavonoids (or bioflavonoids), including about four thousand compounds that are responsible for the colors of fruits and flowers, are believed to have both antioxidant and anti-inflammatory activity. You may read about specific classes of flavonoids, including flavonols, flavones, flavanols, procyanidins, and anthocyanin pigments, and we are learning what each of these compounds does to boost optimal health.

Hosts of experiments on flavonoids found in the soft white skin of citrus fruits (oranges, lemons, grapefruit, and limes) have suggested that these key nutrients increase immune system activation. Other good sources of flavonoids include apricots, cherries, grapes, black currants, blackberries, papayas, green peppers, broccoli, eggplants, squash, tomatoes, tea, red wine, and parsley.

Quercetin, the most abundant flavonoid in apples, has been found to modify inflammatory responses by inhibiting the release of prostaglandins, an inflammatory compound that results in pain. Some studies indicate that quercetin may benefit those with *gout* (a form of arthritis) because it inhibits uric acid production in a similar way as the drug allopurinol. The skin of apples contains the mineral boron, which is key in preventing calcium loss and helps protect against *osteoporosis* (brittle bones). Apples are also rich in the soluble fiber pectin, which helps fill you up so you don't snack.

A study performed at Cornell University revealed that one apple has about 450 milligrams of phytochemicals, which include flavonoids, phenolic compounds, and vitamin C. Researchers at Cornell suggest there is a synergistic antioxidant between these phytochemicals that makes them far more effective than vitamin C alone.

5. These foods are **immunity boosters.** Because some types of pain problems are caused when the immune system goes haywire, it makes good sense to do all you can to keep your immune system functioning at its peak. Many foods recommended in the Pain-Free Diet are high in the mineral zinc to help boost immunity. The plant-based and dairy foods are filled with the necessary calcium and magnesium to build strong bones and relax tense muscles. Magnesium-rich foods such as nuts help to keep muscles supple and prevent aches and pains. In addition, coumarins, nutrients found in limes, carrots and oranges, help keep the immune system healthy. Lycopenes, found in the red pigment of tomatoes and red grapefruit, may also boost your body's immune function and have an anti-inflammatory affect in the body. Garlic, onions, mustard, turmeric, and ginger are also anti-inflammatory.

Pain-Free Super Foods

- **BLACK CHERRIES** contain antioxidants.
- **BLACKBERRIES** have salicylic acid, which is the same active ingredient in aspirin.
- **BROCCOLI** is a powerful antioxidant. It contains vitamin C and calcium.
- **CHEESE (DAIRY AND SOY)** contains calcium for stronger bones. Strong bones are important to prevent osteoporosis and fractures.
- **CHILE PEPPERS** are filled with capsaicin, which gives food a spicy kick and fights inflammation. The hotter the food, the more capsaicin, and the greater the benefit.
- **CURRY, GINGER, MUSTARD, AND TURMERIC,** which contain curcumin, an anti-inflammatory.
- **GREEN TEA** (or black tea that contains theaflavins) has strong phytochemicals that help protect the body. They short-circuit the process that leads to inflammation.
- **OLIVE OIL** forms chemicals in the body that decrease inflammation.
- **OMEGA-3 FATTY ACIDS** can decrease inflammation. Such fish as salmon, sardines, and tuna are good sources.

- **PINEAPPLE** contains bromelain, an enzyme that helps reduce inflammation.
- **RED GRAPES** contain resveratrol, which protects against coronary disease and cancer, and antioxidants.
- **SOY MILK** may decrease pain. It is low in saturated fat, and tofu is an excellent meat substitute.
- **SWEET POTATOES** reduce C-reactive protein, the inflammation-causing cytokine.
- **WALNUTS** contain vitamin B$_6$ for healthy nerve/cell communication.

HOW THE SUPER FOODS WORK

Fruits and Vegetables

Berries Block Free Radicals

The vitamin C in "purple" berries helps to strengthen the immune system and is important in producing connective tissue, especially collagen. But dark berries such as blueberries, blackberries, cherries, and raspberries also help to ease pain because they are filled with anthocyanins, special chemical components that give the intense color to so many fruits and vegetables. It is thought that these plant compounds sweep out harmful free-radical molecules that trigger inflammation.

In a revealing study at the Western Human Nutrition Research Center in Davis, California, researchers had volunteers eat a bowl of forty-five fresh Bing cherries and then measured the C-reactive protein levels in their blood three hours later. After three hours, all the volunteers' blood levels of C-reactive protein dramatically decreased. Researchers concluded that some chemical (anthocyanins) specific to this fruit had an anti-inflammatory effect in the body.

As an extra bonus, one half cup of blueberries (40 calories) or blackberries (30 calories) has more antioxidant power than five servings of green peas, carrots, apples, squash, or broccoli.

Grapes and Red Wine Block Inflammation and Pain

Some new studies suggest that resveratrol, a natural compound found in more than seventy plants, including grapes and berries, protects against oxidation and fungal infection caused by external stresses such as temperature extremes and ultraviolet light. Resveratrol is found in high concentrations in red wine, though its levels may vary depending on the particular wine. Scientists have identified resveratrol as a powerful antioxidant, more potent than vitamin E, and conclude that it may protect against cancer and heart disease.

While we lack solid evidence showing resveratrol's effectiveness in natural dietary supplements, we do have substantiation that resveratrol works in red wine. Researchers have also found that resveratrol blocks the activation of the COX-2 enzyme, the real culprit in igniting inflammation and pain in the body. Some believe that resveratrol may turn out to be an improvement over aspirin in treating painful diseases associated with COX-2, such as osteoarthritis.

Top Ten Pain-Free Fruits

Wild blueberries

Cranberries

Blackberries

Prunes

Raspberries

Strawberries

Red Delicious apples

Granny Smith apples

Sweet cherries

Black plums

Green and Black Tea Are Super-antioxidants

Some recent studies indicate that the antioxidants in green and black tea are more potent than those found in many fruits and vegetables. Tea also contains powerful anti-inflammatory compounds called polyphenols that have been shown to inhibit the production of nitric oxide, which is involved with inflammation. The best known polyphenol is epigallocatechin-3 gallate (EGCG), a chemical that has been shown to reduce the activity of cyclooxygenase-2 (COX-2), the key inflammatory enzyme in *arthritis*. EGCG has also been shown to promote weight loss in some studies.

Up until now, most research has been done on green tea, although black tea is the most widely consumed worldwide. As I've reviewed the results from medical journals, I believe that black tea has comparable antioxidant activity to green tea. I encourage my patients to drink the tea they most enjoy.

Peppers Reduce Substance P

Sweet bell peppers, as well as spicy chile peppers, are filled with the phytochemical capsaicin, which packs an impressive punch against inflammation. Capsaicin reduces levels of substance P, the compound in the body that triggers inflammation and pain impulses from the central nervous system. It is also thought that this pain-relieving phytochemical triggers the body to release endorphins, nature's own opiates. Red peppers are also filled with salicylates, which are aspirin-like compounds.

Pineapple Promotes Healing

For years, I've recommended pineapple to athletes on my soccer team to help heal sports injuries. The reason is bromelain, the key enzyme in pineapple that works in the body by inhibiting the release of certain inflammation-causing chemicals. Some studies show that bromelain enzymes can help reduce pain with osteoathritis. Pineapple also has manganese, a bone-building mineral, and vitamin C, which helps to strengthen collagen.

Spice It Up!

THERE ARE MANY herbs that reduce inflammation in the body if used regularly. For instance, ginger is a strong anti-inflammatory and has been shown in scientific studies to ease arthritis pain. Chile peppers contain capsaicin, which is used in a variety of over-the-counter rubs and salves to help relieve muscle aches and pain. Studies show that capsaicin works by reducing substance P, a neuropeptide that is found at nerve endings and is involved in transmitting the pain signal to the brain. Some of my patients also find benefit in taking cayenne and ginger capsules found at any supermarket or natural foods store.

By sprinkling turmeric, which contains curcumin, into your favorite dishes, you could help to stop pain in its tracks. Experts credit curcumin's anti-inflammatory effects for its ability to stop pain. Curcumin is added to many Indian dishes, as turmeric is the main ingredient in curry powder. You can use turmeric with rice, lentils, and other vegetables, or sprinkle it on your salad for a burst of color. Mustard also contains curcumin, and may be used in cooking and dining in such forms as mustard greens, the prepared mustard condiment, mustard powder, and mustard seeds.

Whole Grains and Complex Carbs

B Vitamins Act as Pain Relievers

If your current diet is heavy in sugar, refined flour, coffee, and alcohol, you may have reduced stores of B vitamins in your body. Some new research points to B vitamins in complex carbohydrates as being important in ending pain, particularly nociceptive pain, which comes when you have a sprain, fracture, bump, bruise, inflammation from infection or arthritic disorder, and myofascial pain (abnormal muscle stresses). Previous studies explored the possibility that the effects of vitamin B_1 (thiamin), B_6 (pyridoxine), and B_{12} (cyanocobalamin) might reduce inflammation. The new findings, presented at the American Physiological Society Conference in San Diego, California, concluded that some B vitamins may be clinically effective in treating painful conditions such as lumbago, sciatica, and other types of pain by acting as an analgesic (pain reliever).

Findings from the National Institutes of Health link vitamin B_3 (niacin or niacinamide) with improved range of motion and reduced pain and inflammation. It is thought that vitamin B_3 may be helpful in preventing osteoarthritis by enhancing glucocorticoid secretion (natural steroid), which would decrease inflammation in the body.

Foods high in B vitamins include brown rice, lentils, chickpeas, spinach, black beans, kidney beans, oranges, broccoli, peanuts, walnuts, soybeans, and fish.

Boost Bones and Weight Loss with Dairy

ALONG WITH THE wide selection of fruits, vegetables, whole grains, legumes, and nuts and seeds, you will also take advantage of the many benefits of fat-free and low-fat dairy products, such as low-fat milk, buttermilk, cheese and cheese products, cottage cheese, ice milk, and yogurt. Not only does the calcium from dairy help to keep bones strong, some research indicates that dairy foods promote weight loss by breaking down the fat in cells. Studies also show that a diet high in low-fat dairy products and fruits and vegetables significantly lowers blood pressure.

Dietary Fiber Keeps You Full

We know that high-fiber diets decrease the risk of some types of cancer and make it easier to maintain a normal weight. The American Dietetic Association recommends 25 to 35 grams of dietary fiber per day. With the Pain-Free

Diet, you get *in excess of 40* grams of dietary fiber per day, helping you to feel full and keeping your blood sugar levels balanced.

There are different types of fiber. Soluble fiber is found in oats, barley, beans, apples, and oranges, among other grains, fruits, and vegetables. This type of fiber helps to lower blood cholesterol and improve blood sugar control in those with diabetes. Studies have found a 28 percent reduction in C-reactive protein levels (pro-inflammatory markers) when study volunteers consumed a whole-food vegan diet rich in soluble fiber. Insoluble fiber, found in whole wheat bread and brown rice, has a major impact upon gastrointestinal transit time. In my practice, patients who eat a diet high in fiber find that it's easier to be compliant to the diet because they feel full. To include more fiber in your diet, consider the following tips:

- Select more legumes that are very high in fiber, such as red beans, black beans, and great northern beans.
- Eat raw vegetables for snacks. Two carrots will give you a day's supply of vitamin A and provide more than 7 grams of fiber.
- Read the cereal box ingredients label at the supermarket. If the cereal has less than 3 grams of fiber, put it back on the shelf.
- Add dried fruits to your cereal. For instance, three prunes can give you 4 grams of fiber.
- Keep your vegetables crisp—not mushy—when you cook them. Eat fruits and vegetables with skins on, to boost the fiber content.

Whole Grains Boost Weight Loss

For years, the top diets have all but banned whole grains, thinking that these carbohydrates would cause a sudden spike and then fall in blood sugar, and result in increased hunger and weight gain. Now we know that whole grains, including some breakfast cereals (bran flakes and shredded wheat), brown rice, barley, bran, bulgur, and oatmeal, actually help keep blood sugar levels steady, helping to reduce the risk of metabolic syndrome, which is associated with pro-inflammatory markers in the body. Several large studies have also shown that intake of whole grains, as opposed to refined grains, is inversely associated with weight gain and body fat distribution.

Whole-grain foods are high in fiber and water content. It is thought that whole grains may protect against weight gain through several mechanisms that involve effects on satiety (feeling of being full), glucose and insulin responses, and antioxidant properties.

Nondairy Foods That Are High in Calcium

YOU WILL GET plenty of calcium from nondairy foods, such as legumes, soy nuts, calcium-fortified soy milk, artichokes, beet greens, broccoli, brussels sprouts, cabbage, celery, carrots, collards, kale, lima beans, snap beans, spinach, and Swiss chard. Not only is broccoli lower in calories and high in phytonutrients, it one of the highest amounts of calcium among vegetables, with over 60 milligrams of calcium for one cup of cooked broccoli (or as much calcium as 2 ounces of low-fat milk).

Whole grains include all three parts of the grain kernel—the bran, germ, and endosperm—and are excellent sources of vitamins and minerals such as thiamin, riboflavin, niacin, vitamin E, magnesium, phosphorus, selenium, zinc, and iron. One slice of sprouted wheat bread, ½ cup of cooked brown rice, 2 ounces of cooked oatmeal, ½ cup of dry whole-grain cereal, or ½ cup of cooked whole-grain pasta equals one serving that is packed with fiber.

Unlike many weight-loss plans, to the Pain-Free Diet urges you to include at least two servings of whole grains during the Weight Loss level, and three servings once you enter the Lifelong level, selecting foods whose first ingredient contains the word *whole* instead of *enriched*.

Whole grains need twice as much water or liquid as regular grains (except for quick-cooking brown rice), and do not cook instantly. You can soak the grain overnight to reduce the cooking time. This works well with oats or brown rice.

Anytime Foods—Anytime You Need Them

SURE, THERE WILL be moments when you are simply starving. Or at least that's what you think at the time. That's why you need to keep plenty of "anytime foods" on hand. These are listed on page 109, and include such foods as cabbage, celery, and lettuce (all of which have virtually no calories). I have several patients who regularly have a large bowl of sautéed or raw red and green cabbage midafternoon if they are unusually hungry. Another patient snacks on celery sticks in his cubicle at work, and most patients thrive on eating a large bowl of *Dr. McIlwain's Anytime Vegetable Soup* (page 139), which can be consumed *anytime* you are hungry. Cucumbers and pickles are also included in the anytime foods. If you have a sweet tooth, try the new bread-and-butter pickles that are sweetened without sugar. Delicious!

Protein, Nuts, and Fats

Good Fats Reduce Inflammatory Markers

Remember the time when *fat* was a negative word? Those who stayed on a very low-fat diet missed out on a lot of delicious food such as nuts and seeds, olives, and avocados—not to mention the health benefits these foods provide.

I believe that *fat* can be a superhealthy word. On the Pain-Free Diet, you are encouraged to add fat to your diet, specifically the monounsaturated fat that comes from olive oil, canola oil, peanut oil, olives, and avocados, among other foods. Monounsaturated fats help reduce insulin resistance, which is important in weight loss and also in decreasing pro-inflammatory markers in your body.

You will also enjoy a host of foods filled with polyunsaturated fatty acids (PUFAs) such as omega-3s in salmon, sardines, tuna, walnuts, flaxseed or flaxseed oil, and soy-based foods. Omega-3 fatty acids increase production of inhibitory prostaglandins which help reduce inflammatory markers in the body. In animal studies, rats with arthritis that were fed diets rich in the omega-3 fatty acid eicosapentaenoic acid (EPA), fared better with pain control than did control animals. Other studies show that when people affected by inflammatory arthritis are given omega-3 fatty acids, the pain and stiffness are reduced.

Dietary sources of omega-3 fatty acids include fish oils and some plant and nut oils. Nuts such as English walnuts and vegetable oils such as soybean, flaxseed, linseed, and canola contain alpha-linolenic acid (ALA). Flaxseed, in particular, contains a combination of omega-3 and omega-6 fatty acids, along with fiber—all important in the Pain-Free Diet. You can easily add flaxseed oil in the recommended Berry Nice Smoothie (page 113).

In Western diets, most people eat about ten times more omega-6 fatty acids than omega-3 fatty acids. The large amounts of omega-6 fatty acids come from vegetable oils (corn, soybean, sunflower, wheat germ, and sesame oils) that contain linoleic acid. In the body, omega-6 and omega-3 fatty acids compete to be converted to active metabolites. We now realize that too much omega-6 (or too little omega-3) results in inflammation. It's important to balance the intake of omega-6 and omega-3 fatty acids.

Legumes Fill You Up and Prevent Overeating

Legumes (beans, lentils, and peas) are also high in phytochemicals and have been called the "meat for vegetarians" for decades. Filled with carbohydrates, protein, and soluble dietary fiber, legumes have resistant starch that does not digest easily and which helps slow the rate at which glucose (blood sugar) enters your bloodstream. Resistant starch goes past the stomach and small intestine before settling in the colon. Because of this action, legumes fill you up, keep your blood glucose levels even, and help prevent hunger pangs that cause you to overeat.

Some new studies reveal that legumes are rich in healing antioxidants, and black beans come out on top, followed by red, brown, yellow, and white beans. One particular class of compounds, the anthocyanins, are particularly abundant in legumes. In fact, the levels of anthocyanins in black beans are ten times greater than the overall antioxidants found in oranges. In some studies, anthycyanins have been found to have the strongest anti-inflammatory effect of any flavonoid tested.

Beans Fill You Up

BEANS ARE NATURALLY low in fat and calories and high in fiber and protein. Just ½ cup of beans has 20 to 120 calories, 2 to 5 grams of fiber, and 2 to 11 grams of protein.

Nuts Contain Anti-inflammatory Compounds

Nuts are a super source of magnesium, vitamin E, and omega-3 fatty acids. For example, peanuts contain resveratrol, the potent anti-inflammatory phytoestrogen found in red grapes and red wine. Peanut butter and other nut butters have no trans fats and are great protein substitutes. Some new findings indicate that pine nuts have a fatty acid that releases an appetite-suppressing hormone called cholecystokinin (CKK). If this is proven, imagine snacking on some pine nuts before dinner and then feeling full after eating just half of your meal.

The only drawback to nuts is the calorie count—it is relatively high. For example, one ounce of peanuts is about 165 calories. Two tablespoons of natural peanut butter is 190 calories. While I encourage you to include nuts in your diet, it's also important to keep track of the serving size, as I have done in the suggested menus on pages 103 to 143.

Protein Helps Control Hunger

The diverse protein choices on the Pain-Free Diet will keep you full and compliant to the plan. Initially, you will eat more protein-rich foods like eggs and fish and limit your complex carbohydrates to help control hunger and cravings, which will get you started losing weight. Then after two weeks at the Jump Start level, you will add more complex carbohydrates (low-starch vegetables, super-antioxidant fruits, and whole grains) to give you a steady weight loss.

As an example, breakfast most mornings on the first two levels will be some type of egg recipe, using whole eggs, egg whites, and egg substitutes. Eggs are loaded with an essential amino acid called leutine, which provides a weight-loss advantage during dieting by helping to reduce loss of lean tissue, promote loss of body fat, and stabilize blood glucose levels. Eggs help to maintain lean muscle mass which is crucial for long-term weight loss (muscle burns fat and calories).

Fish is another low-calorie, high protein mainstay of this diet plan. Some fish, such as salmon, tuna, and trout, are filled with omega-3 fatty acids. Marine omega-3 fatty acids contain eicosapentaenoic acid (EPA) and docosa-hexaenoic acid (DHA), which are known to decrease inflammation in the body, resulting in reduced pain.

Human studies with marine omega-3 fatty acids show a direct relationship between increased DHA consumption and diminished C-reactive protein levels (reduced inflammation). Findings also indicate that women who eat fish twice weekly have half the risk of getting inflammatory arthritis as women who eat only one serving per week. (Some plant foods are also sources of omega-3 fatty acids, including walnuts, tofu and soybean products, flaxseed and flaxseed oil, and canola oil.)

Top Ten Pain-Free Protein Sources

1. Fish
2. Eggs (whole eggs, egg whites, egg substitutes)
3. Soy products
4. Legumes
5. Low-fat dairy products
6. Nuts, seeds, and soy nuts
7. Peanut butter and nut butters
8. Veggie burgers
9. Black bean burgers
10. High-protein pasta

Soy's Isoflavones Lead to Lean Bodies

I recommend the use of soy-based products in the Pain-Free Diet. Soy products are dairy free and do not contain saturated fat. They also have special phytonutrients called isoflavones, compounds in plant foods that are converted into phytoestrogens (plant estrogens that are close in structure to the body's form of estrogen). As an added benefit, researchers have found increased metabolism and significantly decreased body weights and adipose (fatty) tissue disposition in those who eat a diet high in soy isoflavones. We now believe that decreased weight and body fat favor the production of *less inflammatory activity*, which is a *bonus* for those with pain.

On page 106, I will give you a list of soy-based products to choose from—many are conveniently located in your grocer's freezer or produce section.

Reduce Saturated and Trans Fats in Your Pain-Free Diet

CHANGE THIS:	TO THIS:
Ice cream	Ice milk, sherbet, frozen yogurt, frozen soy confection
Butter	No-trans-fats spread
Whole milk	Low-fat, skimmed, or soy milk
Creamed soups	Low-fat variety and skimmed milk
French fries	Baked oven fries
Potato chips	Baked crackers or pretzels
Cream	Evaporated skim milk, soy milk
Fried chicken	Soy chicken or baked chicken (no skin)
Spaghetti sauce with meat	Tomato sauce, fresh tomatoes with herbs
Hamburger	Sandwich of soy "chicken" or skinless chicken
Candy bar	Fruit or nuts
Grilled cheese sandwich	Whole-grain bread with low-fat or soy cheese
Omelet	Egg substitutes or egg whites
Pancakes, biscuits, muffins	Whole-grain English muffins
Pound cake	Angel food cake
Regular mayonnaise	Low-fat or soy mayonnaise

Watch for This Product

DOLCE FUTURO-SWEET FUTURE is a premium light ice cream with 50 percent less fat, 50 percent fewer calories, and 80 percent less sugar than regular ice cream. It has no added sugar, is high in fiber, gluten free, and egg yolk free, in addition to being packaged in 3-ounce portion-control cups (60 calories). This controlled-calorie snack will be available in most grocery stores by 2007.

The Glycemic Index

Most of the recommended foods in the Pain-Free Diet rank low on the glycemic index (GI). The glycemic index is a numerical system that ranks carbohydrates on a scale of 0 to 100, according to their effect on blood glucose levels. In Harvard studies, scientists measured the amount of sugar that different foods released in their body right after they were ingested. Foods that gave a sugar "boost" appeared to increase weight gain and obesity, as well as added to the risk of getting heart disease and diabetes. These studies reported that foods pure in protein and fat (such as meat, chicken, and fish) have a glycemic index of zero. Contrary to these foods, a baked potato has a glycemic index of 85. A food low on the glycemic index (meat, chicken, fish, soy products, and some vegetables) will cause a small rise in blood sugar; a food high on the glycemic index (baked potato, doughnuts, pastries, and other high-starch foods) will trigger a more dramatic rise, which can cause an increase in appetite and boost in pro-inflammatory markers.

Select Foods Low on the Glycemic Index:
Nonstarchy vegetables
Soy products, nuts, seeds, and legumes
Whole-grain breads, especially those that contain whole seeds
Whole-grain pastas
Wheat bran, barley, brown rice, and oats
Low-fat dairy
Fruits such as apples, cherries, grapes, pears, strawberries, and blueberries

Avoid Foods High on the Glycemic Index:
White potatoes
Refined grains, such as white flour and white rice

Vegetables high in starch (corn)
Pastries and cookies
Candy

SELECTING PAIN-FREE SUPPLEMENTS

Your body needs certain vitamins and minerals to make and maintain your joints' normal collagen and cartilage structures. These include vitamins A, B_5, B_6, zinc, boron, and copper. Also, scientists theorize that when tissue stores of selenium are depleted in the body, immunity is impaired. If you have frequent pain, you may benefit from supplements of selenium, an essential trace element, which reduces the production of inflammatory prostaglandins and leukotrienes. Selenium also fights viruses by helping boost T-cell counts in the immune system. You can get adequate amounts of these and other important vitamins and minerals by taking a daily vitamin-mineral supplement.

I also believe it's important to take a few natural dietary supplements, particularly those that are known to decrease inflammation in the body, such as the marine omega-3 fatty acids, which contain EPA and DHA. For example, just one 1,000 milligram capsule of omega-3 fish oil provides about the same amount of valuable marine fatty acids as four ounces of salmon. Vegetarians and vegans who do not want to eat fish or take a fish oil supplement can gain this anti-inflammatory benefit with borage seed oil, flaxseed oil, black currant seed oil, or evening primrose oil—all reported to be helpful in offsetting inflammation in the body.

Here are a few more herbs and supplements that may be helpful:

Boswellia is an herb that blocks pro-inflammatory chemicals called leukotrienes and improves the blood supply to joint tissue.

White willow bark is another botanical with aspirinlike qualities similar to nonsteroidal anti-inflammatory drugs that inhibit the system's pro-inflammatory cytokines.

Feverfew is said to reduce inflammation as well as prostaglandins. In fact, Canada's Health Protection Branch recognizes feverfew as a nonprescription drug for preventing headaches or migraines.

Ginger reduces inflammation and symptoms of osteoarthritis, in clinical studies. In one study, 63 percent of the patients with osteoarthritis of the knee who took ginger reported reduced pain in the knee while standing and less pain after walking fifty feet. Ginger has also been used to treat migraine headache.

Turmeric, a member of the ginger family, protects the body against the ravages of oxygen free radicals and has a potent anti-inflammatory compound called curcumin.

Nettle contains a variety of natural chemicals, such as cyclooxygenase and lipooxygenase, that may slow the enzymes that trigger inflammation. In fact, nettle leaf has been used for years in Germany as a safe treatment of arthritis. In a study published in the *Journal of the Royal Society of Medicine*, researchers applied stinging nettle leaves to the hands of twenty-seven arthritis sufferers. After one week, they found that stinging nettles not only significantly reduced pain, but also that the level of that pain stayed lower through most of the treatment. They concluded that nettles contain serotonin and histamine, both neurotransmitters that affect pain perception and transmission at the nerve endings.

Valerian is another botanical that is safe and effective when taken right before bedtime, if you have trouble falling asleep.

Glucosamine, a naturally occurring amino sugar found in human joints and connective tissues, is useful in maintaining lubrication in the joints, stimulating cartilage repair chemistry, and slowing the breakdown of cartilage.

I'd like you to consider taking one or more of the following Pain-Free dietary supplements. All of these supplements complement the anti-inflammatory foods discussed in this step. You may want to take a multivitamin without iron, a calcium with vitamin D supplement, marine omega-3 fatty acids, flaxseed oil supplements, and glucosamine. Or you might find that your diet is extremely nutritious now and may choose to take only a few supplements that are known to decrease inflammation, such as bromelain and ginger. Whatever you decide, I recommend that you always check with your doctor before taking any natural dietary supplement, just to make sure it is safe in your situation.

- Multivitamin without iron
  Dosage: 1 daily
- Calcium with vitamin D
  Dosage: Supplement your diet to ensure 1,000–1,500 total mg daily with food and natural supplements
- Marine omega-3 fatty acids (fish oil)
  Dosage: 1–2 g daily
- Flaxseed oil (capsule)
  Dosage: 1 g daily
- Bromelain (capsule)
  Dosage: 200–300 mg, three times daily (1 hour before meals)
- Quercetin or other citrus flavonoids
  Dosage: 500 mg, twice daily (with meals)
- Boswellia (herb)
  Dosage: Follow package instructions
- Ginger (herb)
  Dosage: Follow package instructions
- White Willow Bark (herb)
  Dosage: Follow package instructions
- Feverfew (herb)
  Dosage: Follow package instructions
- Nettle (herb)
  Dosage: Follow package instructions
- Valerian (herb)
  Dosage: 400–800 mg in supplement form, ½ hour before bedtime
- Glucosamine
  Dosage: 500 mg, three times daily

Putting it into Practice

REMEMBER FRANK, THE patient who had lost weight repeatedly on a variety of popular diets but always gained it back? Frank was a "diet expert." He was highly successful on the Cybervision diet, Physicians' Weight-Loss plan, Richard Simmons's Deal-a-Meal, the Atkins diet, and the South Beach diet. Yet each time he lost weight, he invariably gained it back again. Frank felt hopeless about his weight and its negative health consequences until he started the Pain-Free Diet.

There is no denying that many popular diets can help you lose weight if you stick with the program. But I want you to do more than simply lose weight. I want you to keep it off. I want you also to change your body chemistry by reducing the pro-inflammatory markers along with the pounds. In short, I want your pain to go away for good. You can only do that by permanently eliminating your excess weight and belly fat.

In this section of *Diet for a Pain-Free Life*, you will learn how to easily implement the Pain-Free Diet into your daily lifestyle. I've given you a sample 28-day program of delicious menus with recipes, lists of foods to choose from as you create your own meal plan, plus daily reminders of when to use moist heat, exercise, and relax (see Rx #2).

Before you begin, write your height and weight in the appropriate spaces on page 73. I then want you to use this information to calculate your body mass index, using the chart on page 69, so you can assess whether you are overweight or obese. You will also need a tape measure to take your hip and waist measurements, to calculate your hip/waist ratio (page 70)—a key measurement that can indicate the presence of inflammation in the body.

CALCULATING YOUR BODY MASS INDEX

The body mass index (BMI) is a ratio of an individual's height and weight, and can often determine if the person is overweight or obese. For this program's purpose, I'd like you to keep track of your BMI each week to measure your weight-loss progress.

To calculate your BMI, you can use this formula:

$$BMI = \frac{\text{weight in pounds} \times 703}{\text{height in inches}^2}$$

Or, consult the height-weight chart on page 69.

Once you've found your BMI then, look at the following assessment chart. If your BMI is between 25 and 30, you are considered overweight; if it is above 30, you are considered obese. For instance, if you are 5' 5" tall and weigh 151 pounds, you are considered to be "overweight." If you are the same height and weigh 180 pounds, you are in the "obese" category. If you are 5' 11", you are overweight at 179 pounds, and obese at 215 pounds. Again, as I have discussed, being overweight or obese is associated with increased levels of pro-inflammatory markers.

The BMI is used by many health-care practitioners; however, it can be misleading in some adults, especially men and women who have large frames or an abundance of muscle. Even though these men and women may have a BMI over 25, they might not have excessive body fat.

BMI	WEIGHT STATUS
Below 18.5	Underweight
18.6–24.9	Normal
25.0–29.9	Overweight
30.0 and above	Obese

	4'5"	4'6"	4'7"	4'8"	4'9"	4'10"	4'11"	5'0"	5'1"	5'2"	5'3"	5'4"	5'5"	5'6"	5'7"	5'8"	5'9"	5'10"	5'11"	6'0"	6'1"	6'2"	6'3"	6'4"	6'5"	6'6"	6'7"	6'8"	6'9"	6'10"
330	83	80	77	74	71	69	67	64	62	60	59	57	55	53	52	50	49	47	46	45	44	42	41	40	39	38	37	36	35	35
320	80	77	74	72	69	67	65	62	60	59	57	55	53	52	50	49	47	46	45	44	42	41	40	39	38	37	36	35	34	33
310	78	75	72	69	67	65	63	61	59	57	55	53	52	50	49	47	46	44	43	42	41	40	39	38	37	36	35	34	33	32
300	75	72	70	67	65	63	61	59	57	55	53	51	50	48	47	46	44	43	42	41	40	39	37	37	36	35	34	33	32	31
290	73	70	67	65	63	61	59	57	55	53	51	50	48	47	46	44	43	42	41	40	39	37	36	35	34	34	33	32	31	30
280	70	67	65	63	61	59	57	55	53	51	50	48	47	45	44	43	41	40	39	38	37	36	35	34	33	32	32	31	30	29
270	68	65	63	61	58	56	55	53	51	49	48	46	45	44	42	41	39	38	37	36	35	34	33	32	32	31	30	30	29	28
260	65	63	60	58	56	54	53	51	49	48	46	45	43	42	41	40	38	37	36	35	34	33	32	32	31	30	29	29	28	27
250	63	60	58	56	54	52	50	49	47	46	44	43	42	40	39	38	37	36	35	34	33	32	31	30	30	29	28	27	27	26
240	60	58	56	54	52	50	48	47	45	44	43	41	40	39	38	36	35	34	33	33	32	31	30	29	28	28	27	26	26	25
230	58	55	53	52	50	48	46	45	43	42	41	39	38	37	36	35	34	33	32	31	30	30	29	28	27	27	26	25	25	24
220	55	53	51	49	48	46	44	43	42	40	39	38	37	36	34	33	32	32	31	30	29	28	28	27	27	26	25	25	24	23
210	53	51	49	47	45	44	42	41	40	38	37	36	35	34	33	31	31	30	29	28	28	27	26	26	25	24	24	23	23	22
200	50	48	46	45	44	42	41	40	38	37	35	34	33	32	31	30	30	29	28	27	26	26	25	24	24	23	22	21	21	21
190	48	46	44	43	41	40	38	37	36	35	34	33	32	31	30	29	28	27	26	26	25	24	24	23	23	22	21	21	20	20
180	45	43	42	40	39	38	36	35	34	33	32	31	30	29	28	27	27	26	25	24	24	23	22	22	21	21	20	19	19	19
170	43	41	40	38	37	36	35	34	33	32	31	30	28	27	27	26	25	24	24	23	22	22	21	21	20	20	19	19	18	18
160	40	39	37	36	35	33	32	31	30	29	28	27	27	26	25	24	23	22	22	21	21	20	19	19	18	18	18	17	17	17
150	38	36	35	34	32	31	30	29	28	27	26	25	24	23	23	22	22	21	20	20	19	19	18	18	17	17	16	16	16	16
140	35	34	33	31	30	29	28	27	26	26	25	24	23	23	22	21	21	20	20	19	18	18	17	17	17	16	16	15	15	15
130	33	31	30	29	27	26	26	25	25	24	23	22	22	21	20	19	19	18	18	17	17	16	16	15	15	15	14	14	14	14
120	30	29	29	27	26	25	24	23	23	22	21	21	20	19	19	18	18	17	17	16	16	15	15	15	14	14	14	13	13	13

ASSESSING YOUR WAIST-TO-HIP MEASUREMENT

A large waist and belly fat are critical measurements that can indicate the presence of chronic inflammation. For example, studies show that a high waist-to-hip ratio (called central fat) indicates higher levels of C-reactive protein, higher tumor necrosis factor, and higher interleukin-6 levels—all pro-inflammatory markers. Relevant studies show that women who have a waist size larger than 35 inches and men who have a waist size larger than 40 inches have three times the risk for diabetes, high blood pressure, and high cholesterol than do adults with smaller waist sizes.

To determine your waist-to-hip ratio, measure your waist in inches at its narrowest point, and then divide this number by your hip measurement in inches at the widest point. For women, the waist-to-hip score should not exceed 0.80; for men, the score should not exceed 0.95.

For instance, if you are a woman with a waist measurement of 32 inches and a hip measurement of 44 inches, your waist-to-hip score is acceptable (less than 0.80):

32 divided by 44 = 0.76

If you are a woman with a waist of 39 inches and hips of 42 inches, your waist-to-hip score is in the danger zone (above 0.80), increasing your risk of inflammation, disease, and pain:

39 divided by 42 = 0.93

If you are a man whose waistline is 33 inches and your hips are 38 inches, your waist-to-hip measurement is in the acceptable zone (less than 0.95):

33 divided by 38 = 0.86

If you are a man whose waistline is 39 inches and hips of 38 inches, your waist-to-hip score is unacceptable (above 0.95):

39 divided by 38 = 1.03

Personal Waist-to-Hip Ratio Worksheet

Waist (in inches) _____ divided by hips (in inches) _____ = _____

No matter what your BMI or waist-to-hip ratio, you can make key changes in the way you eat, relax, exercise, and sleep—changes that can help you to lose weight, reduce your belly fat and inflammation, and subsequently lessen pain.

LEVEL 1 MEAL PLAN:
JUMP START

The first level in the Pain-Free Diet, called **Jump Start**, lasts 2 weeks. The recommended food choices are high in "good" fat and protein (from plants, fish, and eggs) and will jump-start your diet, allowing you to feel full, stay compliant to the Pain-Free Diet plan, and experience weight loss and some reduction of pain within two weeks.

I have listed on page 103–109 the foods that are approved for all levels of the diet. For now, it might be best if you stick with the following menu selections as you begin to change your dietary habits. These meals and snacks are delicious and filling. You can find their recipes in this book, beginning on page 111. Please drink as much tea (green or black) and water as you wish during this and later levels, but avoid coffee and all sugary sweeteners (including honey). If you enjoy drinking tea with milk, be sure to use soy milk, not dairy milk or "nondairy" whiteners, during the Jump Start level.

Along with the sample daily menus, I suggest other important actions you should consider each day to reduce inflammation and pain. For instance, I highly recommend that you start every day with a warm shower, bath, or soak in a Jacuzzi (for a few minutes) followed by the functional fitness exercises (pages 151 to 167). Ideally, you should follow this with at least 10 to 15 minutes of conditioning exercise, selecting the activity you enjoy from the list. I also recommend your taking advantage of your lunch hour to get at least 10 to 15 minutes of conditioning exercise, working toward a total of 30 minutes most days of the week.

Within each sample daily menu, I have added blocks of time in both midmorning and midafternoon for relaxation. Spending just 5 to 10 minutes twice daily with your eyes closed, visualizing tranquil scenes or listening to classical music while blocking all other worries, can make a big difference in how you perceive and address stress, and how you sleep that night. You will be less reactive and have stronger coping skills if you take this time out from the daily grind. If you are at work, wear headphones during the relaxation period and listen to calming music to separate yourself from workplace demands. I also recommend that you take a warm shower, bath, or soak in a Jacuzzi during the evening hours. This moist heat should be again followed by the functional fitness exercises in Rx #2.

During Jump Start, please record your weight and Pain Quotient (see page 26) at the beginning of each week. While it may take days to a few weeks to realize a noticeable benefit from the combination of these four steps—diet, moist heat, exercise, and relaxation—almost *all of my patients* feel immediate relief of pain and stiffness from this regimen. Once you feel relief, do not stop the necessary ritual of moist heat and range-of-motion/stretching exercises. This will keep you limber so you can be more active, keep your joints flexible, and strengthen your muscles.

WEEK 1 WEIGHT _____
WEEK 1 BMI _____
WEEK 1 PAIN QUOTIENT _____

WAKE-UP
◆ *Warm bath/shower/Jacuzzi and functional fitness exercises*
◆ *Conditioning exercise (15 minutes)*

BREAKFAST
Hidden Yolk Scramble
Berry Nice Smoothie

◆ *Relaxation time-out (10 minutes)*

LUNCH
Morningstar Farms veggie burger (or other brand with 125 calories or less),
   with 1 whole wheat bun (under 125 calories), romaine lettuce, red onion
   slices, 2 tomato slices, and 2 teaspoons Dijon or other mustard
¾ cup blueberries or blackberries

◆ *Conditioning exercise (15 minutes)*

SNACK
½ ounce roasted almonds (10–12 nuts)

◆ *Relaxation time-out (10 minutes)*

DINNER
Sea Bass with Toasted Almonds in a Light Lemon Sauce
Dr. McIlwain's Salad Supreme with Olive Oil Vinaigrette Spritz
¾ cup berries

EVENING
◆ *Warm bath/shower/Jacuzzi and functional fitness exercises*

EVENING SNACK
1 tablespoon peanut butter
1 apple, sliced

DAY 1

DAY 2

WAKE-UP
- *Warm bath/shower/Jacuzzi and functional fitness exercises*
- *Conditioning exercise (15 minutes)*

BREAKFAST
Cheesy Sausage Omelet
¾ cup berries

- *Relaxation time-out (10 minutes)*

LUNCH
1 cup low-fat cottage cheese with ½ cup chopped red and green bell pepper, 2 tablespoons chopped green onion, and ½ tomato, chopped (or substitute ½ cup pineapple chunks)
5 whole-grain crackers

- *Conditioning exercise (15 minutes)*

SNACK
½ ounce roasted almonds (10–12 nuts)

- *Relaxation time-out (10 minutes)*

DINNER
Broiled Tuna Steak with Porcini Mushrooms and Baby Bok Choy
Field, Forest, and Pond Salad
1 cup steamed broccoli florets

EVENING
- *Warm bath/shower/Jacuzzi and functional fitness exercises*

EVENING SNACK
Berry Nice Smoothie

WAKE-UP
- *Warm bath/shower/Jacuzzi and functional fitness exercises*
- *Conditioning exercise (15 minutes)*

BREAKFAST

½ cup old-fashioned oats, toasted, mixed with 1 cup low-fat yogurt

- *Relaxation time-out (10 minutes)*

LUNCH

Robust Vegetarian Chili
¾ cup blueberries

- *Conditioning exercise (15 minutes)*

SNACK

4 sticks celery stuffed with 1 tablespoon peanut butter (total)

- *Relaxation time-out (10 minutes)*

DINNER

1 serving whole-grain pasta (such as Barilla PLUS high-protein pasta) tossed with Thai Peanut Sauce and 2 cups steamed broccoli, cut into bite-size pieces
2 cups romaine lettuce with Olive Oil Vinaigrette Spritz

EVENING
- *Warm bath/shower/Jacuzzi and functional fitness exercises*

EVENING SNACK

Berry Nice Smoothie

DAY 3

DAY 4

WAKE-UP
- *Warm bath/shower/Jacuzzi and functional fitness exercises*
- *Conditioning exercise (15 minutes)*

BREAKFAST
Spanish Omelet
¾ cup berries

- *Relaxation time-out (10 minutes)*

LUNCH
6 ounces tuna, ½ cup mixed arugula, watercress, and sprouts , plus 1 slice avocado, in ½ pita pocket

- *Conditioning exercise (15 minutes)*

SNACK
½ ounce soy nuts mixed with 1 tablespoon dried cranberries

- *Relaxation time-out (10 minutes)*

DINNER
Indian Rocks Broiled Seafood Kabobs
Dr. McIlwain's Salad Supreme with Olive Oil Vinaigrette Spritz
½ cup pineapple chunks

EVENING
- *Warm bath/shower/Jacuzzi and functional fitness exercises*

EVENING SNACK
Berry Nice Smoothie

WAKE-UP
◆ *Warm bath/shower/Jacuzzi and functional fitness exercises*
◆ *Conditioning exercise (15 minutes)*

BREAKFAST
1 Kellogg's Eggo Nutri-Grain Whole Wheat Waffle with 2 teaspoons non-trans-fat spread, ¾ cup berries, and 2 tablespoons light or low-sugar syrup

◆ *Relaxation time-out (10 minutes)*

LUNCH
Morningstar Farms Veggie Burger (or other brand with 125 calories or less) on 1 whole-grain bun (under 125 calories), with romaine lettuce, red onion slices, 2 tomato slices, and 2 teaspoons Dijon or other mustard
¾ cup blueberries

◆ *Conditioning exercise (15 minutes)*

SNACK
1 cup low-fat yogurt

◆ *Relaxation time-out (10 minutes)*

DINNER
So Simple Salmon
Dr. McIlwain's Salad Supreme with Olive Oil Vinaigrette Spritz
Florida Berry Granita

EVENING
◆ *Warm bath/shower/Jacuzzi and functional fitness exercises*

EVENING SNACK
Berry Nice Smoothie

DAY 5

DAY 6

WAKE-UP
◆ *Warm bath/shower and functional fitness exercises*
◆ *Conditioning exercise (15 minutes)*

BREAKFAST
Cheesy Sausage Omelet
¾ cup berries

◆ *Relaxation time-out (10 minutes)*

LUNCH
Vegetarian Chili
Broccolini with Garlic and Ginger
¾ cup berries

◆ *Conditioning exercise (15 minutes)*

SNACK
½ cup Easy Edamame

◆ *Relaxation time-out (10 minutes)*

DINNER
Broiled Divers Scallops (7–8 large scallops) with 2 tablespoons prepared
   cocktail sauce
Dr. McIlwain's Salad Supreme with Olive Oil Vinaigrette Spritz
½ cup steamed asparagus

EVENING
◆ *Warm bath/shower/Jacuzzi and functional fitness exercises*

EVENING SNACK
Berry Nice Smoothie

WAKE-UP
- *Warm bath/shower/Jacuzzi and functional fitness exercises*
- *Conditioning exercise (15 minutes)*

BREAKFAST
Spanish Omelet
¾ cup berries

- *Relaxation time-out (10 minutes)*

LUNCH
6 ounces tuna, ½ cup mixed arugula, watercress, and sprouts, plus 1 slice avocado, in ½ pita pocket

- *Conditioning exercise (15 minutes)*

SNACK
½ ounce soy nuts mixed with 1 tablespoon dried cranberries

- *Relaxation time-out (10 minutes)*

DINNER
Sea Bass with Toasted Almonds in a Light Lemon Sauce
Field, Forest, and Pond Salad
½ cup grapes

EVENING
- *Warm bath/shower/Jacuzzi and functional fitness exercises*

EVENING SNACK
Berry Nice Smoothie

DAY 7

WEEK 2 WEIGHT _____
WEEK 2 BMI _____
WEEK 2 PAIN QUOTIENT_____

WAKE-UP
- ◆ *Warm bath/shower/Jacuzzi and functional fitness exercises*
- ◆ *Conditioning exercise (15 minutes)*

BREAKFAST
Hidden Yolk Scramble
Berry Nice Smoothie

- ◆ *Relaxation time-out (10 minutes)*

LUNCH
2 slices soy cheese (or low-fat or 2% fat cheese) on toasted whole-grain bun
(under 125 calories), with romaine lettuce, red onion slices, 2 tomato
slices, and 1 tablespoon Dijon or other mustard
½ cup pineapple chunks

- ◆ *Conditioning exercise (15 minutes)*

SNACK
½ ounce roasted almonds (10–12 nuts)

- ◆ *Relaxation time-out (10 minutes)*

DINNER
Robust Vegetarian Chili
½ whole-grain pita, spread with 1 teaspoon non-trans-fat margarine and
garlic powder and then toasted
Dr. McIlwain's Salad Supreme with Olive Oil Vinaigrette Spritz

EVENING
- ◆ *Warm bath/ shower/Jacuzzi and functional fitness exercises*

EVENING SNACK
1 apple, sliced
1 tablespoon peanut butter

DAY 8

WAKE-UP
- *Warm bath/shower/Jacuzzi and functional fitness exercises*
- *Conditioning exercise (15 minutes)*

BREAKFAST
   1 Kellogg's Eggo Nutri-Grain Whole Wheat Waffle with 2 teaspoons
      non-trans-fat spread
   ½ cup low-fat yogurt mixed with ½ cup blackberries

- *Relaxation time-out (10 minutes)*

LUNCH
   3 cups steamed vegetables (any combination from page 104)
   ½ cup whole wheat pasta (or Barilla PLUS high-protein pasta) with Thai
      Peanut Sauce
   ½ cup seedless red grapes

- *Conditioning exercise (15 minutes)*

SNACK
   Berry Nice Smoothie

- *Relaxation time-out (10 minutes)*

DINNER
   So Simple Salmon
   Thai Cucumber Salad
   ¾ cup berries

EVENING:
- *Warm bath/shower/Jacuzzi and functional fitness exercises*

EVENING SNACK
   1 apple, sliced
   1 tablespoon peanut butter

DAY 9

DAY 10

WAKE-UP
- *Warm bath/shower/Jacuzzi and functional fitness exercises*
- *Conditioning exercise (15 minutes)*

BREAKFAST
Spanish Omelet
Berry Nice Smoothie

- *Relaxation time-out (10 minutes)*

LUNCH
Morningstar Farms veggie burger (or other brand with 125 calories or less) on 1 whole-grain bun (under 125 calories), with romaine lettuce, red onion slices, 2 tomato slices, and 2 teaspoons Dijon or other mustard
¾ cup blueberries

- *Conditioning exercise (15 minutes)*

SNACK
½ cup Easy Edamame

- *Relaxation time-out (10 minutes)*

DINNER
Grouper with Toasted Almonds in a Light Lemon Sauce
Dr. McIlwain's Salad Supreme with Olive Oil Vinaigrette Spritz
½ cup steamed asparagus

EVENING
- *Warm bath/shower/Jacuzzi and functional fitness exercises*

EVENING SNACK
1 cup low-fat yogurt

WAKE-UP
- *Warm bath/shower/Jacuzzi and functional fitness exercises*
- *Conditioning exercise (15 minutes)*

BREAKFAST
1 cup low-fat yogurt mixed with 2 teaspoons toasted chopped walnuts and ¾ cup blueberries
- *Relaxation time-out (10 minutes)*

LUNCH
6 ounces tuna, ½ cup mixed arugula, watercress, and sprouts, plus 1 slice avocado, in ½ pita pocket
- *Conditioning exercise (15 minutes)*

SNACK
½ ounce soy nuts mixed with 1 tablespoon dried cranberries
- *Relaxation time-out (10 minutes)*

DINNER
Indian Rocks Broiled Seafood Kabobs
Thai Cucumber Salad
1 cup steamed broccoli florets

EVENING
- *Warm bath/shower/Jacuzzi and functional fitness exercises*

EVENING SNACK
¾ cup berries mixed with ½ cup low-fat vanilla yogurt and ½ teaspoon cinnamon.

DAY 11

DAY 12

WAKE-UP
- *Warm bath/shower/Jacuzzi and functional fitness exercises*
- *Conditioning exercise (15 minutes)*

BREAKFAST
    Spanish Omelet
    Florida Berry Granita

- *Relaxation time-out (10 minutes)*

LUNCH
    3 cups steamed vegetables (any combination from page 104)
    ½ cup whole wheat pasta (or Barilla PLUS high-protein pasta) with Thai
        Peanut Sauce

- *Conditioning exercise (15 minutes)*

SNACK
    1 apple, sliced
    1 tablespoon peanut butter

- *Relaxation time-out (10 minutes)*

DINNER
    Broiled fish
    Crispy Apples, Mixed Greens, and Gorgonzola
    ½ cup strawberries

EVENING
- *Warm bath/shower/Jacuzzi and functional fitness exercises*

EVENING SNACK
    Berry Nice Smoothie

WAKE-UP
- *Warm bath/shower/Jacuzzi and functional fitness exercises*
- *Conditioning exercise (15 minutes)*

BREAKFAST
Apples and Oats

- *Relaxation time-out (10 minutes)*

LUNCH
6 ounces albacore tuna tossed with Dr. McIlwain's Salad Supreme with
   Olive Oil Vinaigrette Spritz
½ cup pineapple chunks

- *Conditioning exercise (15 minutes)*

SNACK
½ cup Easy Edamame

- *Relaxation time-out (10 minutes)*

DINNER
Pecan-Crusted Salmon Filets
½ cup cold Multibean Salad tossed with 3 cups (bagged) romaine salad mix
   with Olive Oil Vinaigrette Spritz

EVENING
- *Warm bath/shower/Jacuzzi and functional fitness exercises*

EVENING SNACK
Berry Nice Smoothie

DAY 13

DAY 14

WAKE-UP
- *Warm bath/shower/Jacuzzi and functional fitness exercises*
- *Conditioning exercise (15 minutes)*

BREAKFAST
3–egg white omelet prepared with 1 slice soy or 2%–fat cheese
Berry Nice Smoothie

- *Relaxation time-out (10 minutes)*

LUNCH
Egg and Olive Salad, romaine lettuce, red onion slices, and 2 tomato slices, plus 1 slice avocado in ½ whole-grain pita

- *Conditioning exercise (15 minutes)*

SNACK
1 apple, sliced
1 tablespoon peanut butter

- *Relaxation time-out (10 minutes)*

DINNER
Broiled Tuna Steak with Porcini Mushrooms and Baby Bok Choy
1 cup steamed broccoli and cauliflower medley
½ cup pineapple

EVENING
- *Warm bath/shower/Jacuzzi and functional fitness exercises*

EVENING SNACK
Dessert of your choice from last 2 weeks' menus

LEVEL 2 MEAL PLAN:
WEIGHT LOSS

After following Jump Start successfully for two weeks, you will then begin **Level 2: Weight Loss**. You may remain at this level for weeks or months, depending on how much weight you want to lose. This phase of the Pain-Free Diet has less fat but more complex carbohydrates and protein than Jump Start, so it's guaranteed to keep you feeling full and energetic. It will provide you with approximately 1,400 calories daily. Please continue the moist heat, exercise, and relaxation regimen from the previous level, and note your weight, BMI, and Pain Quotient weekly.

DAY 15

WEEK 3 WEIGHT _____
WEEK 3 BMI _____
WEEK 3 PAIN QUOTIENT _____

WAKE-UP
◆ *Warm bath/shower/Jacuzzi and functional fitness exercises*
◆ *Conditioning exercise (15 minutes)*

BREAKFAST
Scrambled egg sandwich, made with 1 whole egg and 2 whites, 1 toasted
   whole-grain bun (less than 125 calories), and 2 teaspoons trans-fat-free
   margarine
½ cup grapes

◆ *Relaxation time-out (10 minutes)*

LUNCH
1 cup low-fat cottage cheese with ½ cup chopped red and green bell pepper,
   2 tablespoons chopped green onion, and ½ tomato, chopped (or substitute ½ cup pineapple chunks)
5 whole-grain crackers
Florida Berry Granita

◆ *Conditioning exercise (15 minutes)*

SNACK
½ cup Easy Edamame

◆ *Relaxation time-out (10 minutes)*

DINNER
Sea Bass with Toasted Almonds in a Light Lemon Sauce
Field, Forest, and Pond Salad
5 ounces red wine

EVENING:
◆ *Warm bath/shower/Jacuzzi and functional fitness exercises*

EVENING SNACK
Berry Nice Smoothie

WAKE-UP
◆ *Warm bath/shower/Jacuzzi and functional fitness exercises*
◆ *Conditioning exercise (15 minutes)*

BREAKFAST
Spanish Omelet
¾ cup fresh berries

◆ *Relaxation time-out (10 minutes)*

LUNCH
Morningstar Farms veggie burger (or other brand with 125 calories or less)
on 1 whole-grain bun (under 125 calories), with romaine lettuce, red
onion slices, and Dijon or other mustard
Florida Berry Granita

◆ *Conditioning exercise (15 minutes)*

SNACK
½ ounce soy nuts and mixed with 1 tablespoon dried cranberries

◆ *Relaxation time-out (10 minutes)*

DINNER
1 serving whole-grain pasta (such as Barilla PLUS) with Pesto Sauce and 2
cups steamed broccoli, cut into bite-size pieces
2 cups favorite bagged salad with Olive Oil Vinaigrette Spritz
5 ounces red wine

EVENING
◆ *Warm bath/shower/Jacuzzi and functional fitness exercises*

EVENING SNACK
½ cup low-fat vanilla yogurt mixed with ¾ cup berries, and ½ teaspoon
cinnamon,

DAY 16

DAY 17

WAKE-UP
- *Warm bath/shower/Jacuzzi and functional fitness exercises*
- *Conditioning exercise (15 minutes)*

BREAKFAST
1 whole wheat bagel (Sara Lee Heart Healthy or other brand with 220 calories or less) with 2 tablespoons soy cream cheese

- *Relaxation time-out (10 minutes)*

LUNCH
Morningstar Farms soy chicken patty (cut into pieces), tossed with Crispy Apples, Mixed Greens, and Gorgonzola

- *Conditioning exercise (15 minutes)*

SNACK
½ cup low-fat yogurt mixed with ¾ cup berries

- *Relaxation time-out (10 minutes)*

DINNER
Pecan-Crusted Salmon
3 cups romaine lettuce with Olive Oil Vinaigrette Spritz and ½ cup chickpeas
5 ounces red wine

EVENING
- *Warm bath/shower/Jacuzzi and functional fitness exercises*

EVENING SNACK
Berry Nice Smoothie

WAKE-UP
- *Warm bath/shower/Jacuzzi and functional fitness exercises*
- *Conditioning exercise (15 minutes)*

BREAKFAST
Apples and Oats

- *Relaxation time-out (10 minutes)*

LUNCH
Robust Vegetarian Chili
5 whole-grain crackers
¾ cup blueberries

- *Conditioning exercise (15 minutes)*

SNACK
1 apple, sliced
1 tablespoon peanut butter

- *Relaxation time-out (10 Minutes)*

DINNER
Buccaneers' Sloppy Joes, made with 1 toasted whole-grain bun (under 125
   calories), romaine lettuce, 1 slice red onion, and 1 pickle
10 raw baby carrots
5 ounces red wine

EVENING
- *Warm bath/shower/Jacuzzi and functional fitness exercises*

EVENING SNACK
Berry Nice Smoothie

DAY 18

DAY 19

WAKE-UP
- *Warm bath/shower/Jacuzzi and functional fitness exercises*
- *Conditioning exercise (15 minutes)*

BREAKFAST
Cheesy Sausage Omelet
¾ cup strawberries

- *Relaxation time-out (10 minutes)*

LUNCH
Buccaneers' Sloppy Joes (leftovers from day 18) made with 1 toasted whole-grain bun (under 125 calories), romaine lettuce,1 slice red onion slice, and 1 pickle
½ cup pineapple chunks

- *Conditioning exercise (15 minutes)*

SNACK
½ cup Easy Edamame

- *Relaxation time-out (10 minutes)*

DINNER
6 ounces boiled shrimp with 2 tablespoons prepared cocktail sauce
Field, Forest, and Pond Salad
½ cup asparagus
5 ounces red wine

EVENING
- *Warm bath/shower/Jacuzzi and functional fitness exercises*

EVENING SNACK
1 apple, sliced
1 tablespoon peanut butter

WAKE-UP
- *Warm bath/shower/Jacuzzi and functional fitness exercises*
- *Conditioning exercise (15 minutes)*

BREAKFAST
　　1 whole wheat bagel (Sara Lee Heart Healthy or other brand with 220
　　　　calories or less) with 2 tablespoons soy cream cheese

- *Relaxation time-out (10 minutes)*

LUNCH
　　Apple–Butternut Squash Soup
　　1 slice whole-grain bread with 1 slice soy cheese
　　¾ cup blueberries

- *Conditioning exercise (15 minutes)*

SNACK
　　1 apple, sliced
　　1 tablespoon peanut butter

- *Relaxation time-out (10 minutes)*

DINNER
　　So Simple Salmon
　　Florida Orange and Spinach Salad with Sunlight Dressing
　　1 cup steamed broccoli florets
　　5 ounces red wine

EVENING:
- *Warm bath/shower/Jacuzzi and functional fitness exercises*

EVENING SNACK
　　1 cup low-fat vanilla yogurt mixed with ½ cup berries

DAY 20

DAY 21

WAKE-UP
- *Warm Bath/ shower and functional fitness exercises*
- *Conditioning exercise (15 minutes)*

BREAKFAST
1 Kellogg's Eggo Nutri-Grain Whole Wheat Waffle with 1 tablespoon peanut butter and 2 tablespoons low-sugar syrup

- *Relaxation time-out (10 minutes)*

LUNCH
Egg and Olive Salad, 1 cup chopped romaine lettuce, and ½ cup chopped tomato stuffed into ½ whole-grain pita pocket
¾ cup berries topped with 1 tablespoon light Cool Whip

- *Conditioning exercise (15 minutes)*

SNACK
1 low-fat yogurt mixed with ¾ cup berries

- *Relaxation time-out (10 minutes)*

DINNER
Pecan-Crusted Salmon
Florida Orange and Spinach Salad
1 cup steamed vegetable of choice (page 104)
5 ounces red wine

EVENING
- *Warm bath/shower/Jacuzzi and functional fitness exercises*

EVENING SNACK
Dessert of your choice (under 250 calories)

LEVEL 3 MEAL PLAN:
LIFETIME

When you enter the Lifetime level, continue to follow the regimen for **Level 2: Weight Loss**, including fish, eggs, low-fat dairy, and even poultry if you wish, but no meat or processed grains or sugars. You add calories at this point if you can do so without gaining weight. Resume the stricter diet of **Level 1: Jump Start** if you find yourself gaining weight again.

WEEK 4 WEIGHT IN _____

WEEK 4 BMI _____

WEEK 4 PAIN QUOTIENT _____

DAY 22

WAKE-UP
- ◆ *Warm bath/shower and functional fitness exercises*
- ◆ *Conditioning exercise (15 minutes)*

BREAKFAST
1 whole wheat bagel (Sara Lee Heart Healthy or other brand with 220 calories or less), toasted, with 1 tablespoon peanut butter

- ◆ *Relaxation time-out (10 minutes)*

LUNCH
Morningstar Farms soy chicken patty (cut into pieces), tossed with Crispy Apples, Mixed Greens and Gorgonzola

- ◆ *Conditioning exercise (15 minutes)*

SNACK
½ cup blackberries with ½ cup vanilla low-fat yogurt

- ◆ *Relaxation time-out (10 minutes)*

DINNER
Indian Rocks Broiled Seafood Kabobs
Field, Forest, and Pond Salad
5 ounces red wine

EVENING:
- ◆ *Warm bath/shower/Jacuzzi and functional fitness exercises*

EVENING SNACK
Berry Nice Smoothie

WAKE-UP
- ◆ *Warm bath/shower/Jacuzzi and functional fitness exercises*
- ◆ *Conditioning exercise (15 minutes)*

BREAKFAST
Apples and Oats

- ◆ *Relaxation time-out (10 minutes)*

LUNCH
Egg and Olive Salad, 1 cup chopped romaine lettuce, and ½ chopped
    tomato stuffed into ½ whole-grain pita pocket
½ cup pineapple chunks

- ◆ *Conditioning exercise (15 minutes)*

SNACK
½ cup Easy Edamame

- ◆ *Relaxation time-out (10 minutes)*

DINNER
1 serving whole-grain pasta (such as Barilla PLUS) with Pesto Sauce, tossed
    with 2 cups steamed broccoli, cut into bite-size pieces
2 cups favorite bagged salad with Olive Oil Vinaigrette Spritz
5 ounces red wine

EVENING
- ◆ *Warm bath/shower/Jacuzzi and functional fitness exercises*

EVENING SNACK
Berry Nice Smoothie

DAY 23

DAY 24

WAKE-UP
- *Warm bath/shower/Jacuzzi and functional fitness exercises*
- *Conditioning exercise (15 minutes)*

BREAKFAST
Spanish Omelet
1 slice whole-grain toast with 2 teaspoons non-trans-fat spread

- *Relaxation time-out (10 minutes)*

LUNCH
Apple–Butternut Squash Soup
1 slice whole-grain bread with 1 slice 2% swiss cheese melted on top
1 cup french-cut green beans

- *Conditioning exercise (15 minutes)*

SNACK
¾ cup berries
½ cup low-fat vanilla yogurt

- *Relaxation time-out (10 minutes)*

DINNER
6 ounces tuna, water-packed, drained, tossed with Crispy Apples, Mixed
    Greens, and Gorgonzola
5 ounces red wine

EVENING:
- *Warm bath/shower/Jacuzzi and functional fitness exercises*

EVENING SNACK
Berry Nice Smoothie

WAKE-UP
- ◆ *Warm bath/shower/Jacuzzi and functional fitness exercises*
- ◆ *Conditioning exercise (15 minutes)*

BREAKFAST
1 slice whole-grain bread with 1 tablespoon peanut butter (or other nut butter)
Berry Nice Smoothie

- ◆ *Relaxation time-out (10 minutes)*

LUNCH
1 whole-grain bun (under 125 calories), with 2 slices soy cheese (or low-fat
    or 2%–fat cheese), romaine lettuce, 1 slice red onion, 2 slices tomato
½ cup pineapple chunks

- ◆ *Conditioning exercise (15 minutes)*

SNACK
½ ounce smoked almonds (10–12 nuts)

- ◆ *Relaxation time-out (10 minutes)*

DINNER
Almond-Crusted Grouper (use Pecan-Crusted Salmon recipe, substituting
    almonds and grouper)
Dr. McIlwain's Salad Supreme with Olive Oil Vinaigrette Spritz
1 cup steamed vegetable of choice (page 104)
5 ounces red wine

EVENING
- ◆ *Warm bath/shower/Jacuzzi and functional fitness exercises*

EVENING SNACK
Warm Baked Apples and Cinnamon topped with ½ cup low-fat vanilla
    yogurt

DAY 25

DAY 26

WAKE-UP
- *Warm bath/shower/Jacuzzi and functional fitness exercises*
- *Conditioning exercise (15 minutes)*

BREAKFAST
Scrambled egg sandwich, made with 1 whole egg and 2 whites, on a whole-grain bun (under 125 calories), with 2 tablespoons trans-fat-free margarine
½ cup grapes

- *Relaxation time-out (10 minutes)*

LUNCH
Apple–Butternut Squash Soup
1 slice whole grain bread with 1 slice 2%–sharp cheddar cheese melted on top
¾ cup blueberries

- *Conditioning exercise (15 minutes)*

SNACK
½ ounce roasted almonds (10–12 nuts)

- *Relaxation time-out (10 Minutes)*

DINNER
Sea Bass with Toasted Almonds in a Light Lemon Sauce
Dr. McIlwain's Salad Supreme with Olive Oil Vinaigrette Spritz and ½ cup chickpeas
5 ounces red wine

EVENING
- *Warm bath/shower/Jacuzzi and functional fitness exercises*

EVENING SNACK
Warm Cinnamon Apples
½ cup low-fat vanilla yogurt

WAKE-UP
- *Warm bath/shower/Jacuzzi and functional fitness exercises*
- *Conditioning exercise (15 minutes)*

BREAKFAST
Cheesy Sausage Omelet
1 slice whole wheat toast with 2 teaspoons low-sugar jelly

- *Relaxation time-out (10 minutes)*

LUNCH
6 ounces albacore tuna (water-packed, drained) tossed with 2 cups romaine lettuce with Olive Oil Vinaigrette Spritz
1 slice whole wheat bread with 1 slice soy cheese (or low-fat, or 2% fat cheese) melted on top

- *Conditioning exercise (15 minutes)*

SNACK
1 apple, sliced
1 tablespoon peanut butter

- *Relaxation time-out (10 minutes)*

DINNER
Indian Rocks Broiled Seafood Kabobs
3 cups favorite bagged salad with Olive Oil Vinaigrette Spritz
1 cup steamed vegetable of choice (page 104)
5 ounces red wine

EVENING
- *Warm bath/shower/Jacuzzi and functional fitness exercises*

EVENING SNACK
Berry Nice Smoothie

DAY 27

DAY 28

WEEK 5 WEIGHT _____
WEEK 5 BMI: _____
WEEK 5 PAIN QUOTIENT _____

WAKE-UP
◆ *Warm bath/shower/Jacuzzi and functional fitness exercises*
◆ *Conditioning exercise (15 minutes)*

BREAKFAST
1 Kellogg's Eggo Nutri-Grain Whole Wheat Waffle topped with ½ cup
berries and ½ cup low-fat yogurt or soy yogurt

◆ *Relaxation time-out (10 minutes)*

LUNCH
Morningstar Farms veggie burger (or other brand equal to 125 calories or
less) on 1 whole-grain bun (under 125 calories), with romaine lettuce,
red onion slice, and 2 tomato slices
½ cup pineapple chunks

◆ *Conditioning exercise (15 minutes)*

SNACK
Berry Nice Smoothie

◆ *Relaxation time-out (10 minutes)*

DINNER
Broiled Tuna Steak with Porcini Mushrooms and Baby Bok Choy
Crispy Apples, Mixed Greens, and Gorgonzola
1 cup steamed broccoli
5 ounces red wine

EVENING
◆ *Warm bath/shower/Jacuzzi and functional fitness exercises*

EVENING SNACK
Dessert of your choice (under 250 calories)

PAIN-FREE FOOD LISTS WITH SERVING SIZES

Can you modify the menus? Yes! I encourage you to identify the Pain-Free foods and recipes that you enjoy most and use these to create a personalized meal plan. The following lists of Pain-Free foods will be your mainstay while on this diet. With each list, I've given the serving size and the number of servings, depending on your level in the program. Using this wealth of information, you can create a delicious and filling menu that fits your specific taste while following a proven weight-loss program that decreases inflammation and pain.

Pain-Free Foods by Group

Fruits and Vegetables

SUPER-ANTIOXIDANT FRUITS
Level 1: 2–3 servings daily
Level 2: 3–4 servings daily
Level 3: 3–5 servings daily

- Apple, 1 medium
- Apricots, 4 medium
- Banana, ½ medium
- Blackberries, ¾ cup
- Blueberries, ¾ cup
- Boysenberries, ¾ cup
- Cantaloupe, ¼ melon
- Cherries, fresh, 12 large
- Dates, 3 medium
- Figs, dried, 1½ medium
- Grapefruit, ½ large
- Grapes, 18 small
- Honeydew melon, 1 cup cubed
- Kiwi, 1 large
- Mango, ½ small
- Nectarine, 1 small
- Orange, 1 small
- Peach, 1 medium
- Pear, ½ large
- Pineapple, ¾ cup chopped, fresh
- Plum, 2 small
- Pomegranate, ½ medium
- Raisins, 2 tablespoons
- Raspberries, 1 cup
- Strawberries, 1 cup
- Tangelo, 1 large
- Tangerine, 2 small
- Watermelon, 1 cup chopped

Nonstarchy Vegetables

FOR ALL: 1 cup raw or ½ cup cooked = 1 serving
Level 1: 4 servings daily
Level 2: 4–6 servings daily
Level 3: Unlimited servings daily

- Alfalfa sprouts
- Artichokes/artichoke hearts
- Asparagus
- Avocado
- Bamboo shoots
- Bean sprouts
- Beans (green, string, yellow, wax, Italian)
- Broccoli
- Brussels sprouts
- Cabbage
- Carrots
- Cauliflower
- Celery
- Chinese (napa) cabbage
- Cucumber
- Eggplant
- Greens (beet, collard, kale, mustard, turnip)
- Kohlrabi
- Leeks
- Lettuce (endive, escarole, leafy green, romaine, iceberg—also bagged salads with these types of lettuce)
- Mushrooms
- Okra
- Onions
- Parsley
- Snow peas
- Sweet potato (½ medium potato, cooked)
- Peppers (all)
- Radishes
- Rhubarb
- Rutabaga
- Sauerkraut
- Scallions
- Spinach
- Squash (summer)
- Swiss chard
- Tomato (raw, regular, or cherry/grape size, juice, paste, sauce)
- Turnips
- Water chestnuts
- Watercress
- Zucchini

Whole Grains

1 SLICE BREAD = 1 serving
½ CUP COOKED BROWN RICE, OATS, OR WHOLE-GRAIN PASTA = 1 serving
1 OUNCE OF READY-TO-EAT CEREAL OR ½ CUP COOKED CEREAL = 1 serving
    (A product is "whole grain" if the ingredients label says "rye," "whole grain,"
    or "whole wheat.")
Level 1: 2 servings daily
Level 2: 2–3 servings daily
Level 3: 3–5 servings daily

- Barley
- Brown rice
- Buckwheat (kasha)
- Bulgur
- Chickpea flour (gram)
- Couscous
- Millet
- Oats
- Rye
- Soy flour
- Whole wheat bread
- Whole-grain cold cereal (All-Bran, Cheerios, granola, muesli, Grape-nuts, Kashi GoLean, Nutri-Grain, Raisin Bran, shredded wheat, Total, wheat germ, Wheaties)
- Whole-grain hot cereal (muesli, oat bran, oatmeal, Wheatena)
- Wild rice

Proteins, Legumes, and Nuts

FISH: 4 ounces = 1 serving
Level 1: 1–2 servings daily
Level 2: 1–2 servings daily
Level 3: 1–2 servings daily

- Anchovies★
- Atlantic salmon★
- Bass
- Bluefish★
- Catfish
- Capelin (smelts)
- Clam
- Cod
- Crab
- Crawfish
- Dogfish★
- Flounder
- Grouper
- Haddock

▶ Halibut
▶ Lobster
▶ Lox (smoked salmon)
▶ Mackerel★
▶ Mahimahi
▶ Perch
▶ Pike
▶ Pompano
▶ Sardines★
▶ Scallops

▶ Shad★
▶ Shrimp
▶ Striped sea bass
▶ Swordfish
▶ Trout
▶ Tuna (fresh or canned in water)★
▶ Whitefish★
▶ Whiting

★High in omega-3 fatty acids

DRIED BEANS AND PEAS; SOY PRODUCTS
½ cup cooked = 1 serving
1 VEGGIE/GARDEN/SOY BURGER OR VEGETARIAN HOT DOG = 1 serving
Level 1: 2–3 servings daily
Level 2: 2–4 servings daily
Level 3: 2–4 servings daily

▶ Baby lima beans
▶ Black beans
▶ Black-eyed peas
▶ Brown beans
▶ Butter beans
▶ Cannellini beans
▶ Chickpeas
▶ Chili (meatless)
▶ Edamame
▶ Fava beans
▶ Garden burger
▶ Great northern beans
▶ Kidney beans
▶ Lentils (all colors)

▶ Lima beans
▶ Navy beans
▶ Pink beans
▶ Pinto beans
▶ Red beans
▶ Refried, fat-free beans
▶ Soy and soy products (including soy cheeses, yogurts, and other substitutes for dairy; meat substitutes; miso; tempeh; textured soy protein; tofu)
▶ Split peas
▶ Veggie burger
▶ White beans

SEEDS AND NUTS
Level 1: 1–2 servings daily
Level 2: 1–3 servings daily
Level 3: 1– 3 servings daily

- Almonds (11 nuts)
- Almond butter (1 tablespoon)
- Cashew nuts (8 nuts)
- Macadamia nuts (5 nuts)
- Peanuts (12 peanuts)
- Peanut butter (1 tablespoon)

- Pecans (8 nuts)
- Pine nuts (2 tablespoons)
- Pumpkin seeds (½ ounce)
- Sesame seeds (½ ounce)
- Sunflower seeds (½ ounce)
- Walnuts (4 nuts)

DAIRY PRODUCTS
Level 1: 1–2 servings daily
Level 2: 2–3 servings daily
Level 3: 2–3 servings daily

- Milk (fat-free, low-fat, soy)
- Cheese (fat-free, low-fat, soy)
- Cottage cheese (fat-free)
- Cream cheese (fat-free, soy)

- Yogurt (non-fat, low-fat, soy)
- Frozen yogurt (non-fat, low-fat)—limit to ½ cup daily

Oils, Dressings, and Condiments

LIMIT OILS, FAT-FREE MAYONNAISE, DRESSINGS, AND MARGARINE TO A TOTAL OF 3 TEASPOONS DAILY
Level 1: 2 servings daily
Level 2: 1–3 servings daily
Level 3: 2–4 servings daily

- Canola oil (1 teaspoon)
- Fat-free salad dressings (2 teaspoons)
- Fat-free margarine (2 teaspoons)

- Fat-free mayonnaise (2 teaspoons)
- Flaxseed oil (1 teaspoon)
- Olive oil (1 teaspoon)

Beverages

THE FOLLOWING ARE UNLIMITED, EXCEPT FOR WINE:

- Green or black tea (without sugar)
- Decaffeinated coffee (without sugar)
- Diet soft drinks
- Club soda
- Seltzer (plain or flavored, unsweetened)
- Tonic water (artificially sweetened)
- Water
- Red wine (5 ounces a day, Levels 2 and 3 only)

Very Low-Calorie and Unlimited "Anytime" Foods

To succeed with the Pain-Free Diet, it is important to keep low-calorie foods on hand. I recommend storing these foods in snack bags or plastic containers and keeping them with you at work, in the car, and at home. By doing so, you will be less tempted to snack on pro-inflammatory foods or fast foods.

Some of these foods, such as cooked vegetables, taste best when eaten hot. You can prepare these foods ahead of time, store them, and then zap them in the microwave before snacking. Other foods, such as grapes, a plum, or even half a sweet potato, can be eaten cold or at room temperature.

20 TO 40 CALORIES:

Select *one* when you are hungry and dinnertime is an hour away:

¾ cup cooked cauliflower
½ cup whole cranberries (not dried cranberries)
1 cup cooked eggplant
½ cup papaya
¾ cup steamed fresh green beans
1 cup steamed summer squash
1 plum
1 cup kale
5 large green olives

45 TO 65 CALORIES:

Select *one* when you are extremely hungry and it's midafternoon:

1 cup raspberries

1 cup raw or cooked red cabbage

¾ cup diced honeydew melon

¼ cantaloupe

¾ cup pineapple

1 cup grapes

½ baked sweet potato

1 cup watermelon chunks

½ cup green peas

½ pomegranate (approx. 400 seeds)

ANYTIME, UNLIMITED FOODS

All herbs (basil, cilantro, chive, dill, fennel, mint, oregano, rosemary, sage, tarragon, thyme)

All spices (caraway, cayenne, celery seed, chili powder, cinnamon, clove, cumin, curry, nutmeg, pepper, saffron, turmeric)

Braised cabbage

Bread-and-butter pickles (sweetened with Splenda)

Celery

Cucumber

Dill pickles

Dr. McIlwain's Anytime Vegetable Soup (page 139)

Garlic

Ginger

Horseradish

Lemon or lime juice (or zest)

Lettuce (romaine, green leaf, red leaf, iceberg)

Mushrooms

Mustard

Sauerkraut

Spinach

Vanilla

Vinegar (balsamic, rice, wine)

Avoid Foods That Increase Inflammation

On all levels of the Pain-Free Diet, it is important to avoid the following foods, which are known to be pro-inflammatory. Go through your pantry and refrigerator and discard:

Any animal products not listed in the Pain-Free Diet proteins and dairy
   lists (pages 105–107)
Bagels, breads, rolls, muffins, and crackers not made with whole grains
Cakes and pies, except fruit pies
Candy
Cereals that are not labeled "whole grain"
Cookies, unless made with "whole grains"
Corn and cornstarch
Croissants
Doughnuts and other fried pastries
Dressings, shortenings, and spreads that are hydrogenated (not trans-fat-
   free)
Fast food
Fruits in syrup or sugar (frozen or canned)
Gnocchi
Ice cream, sherbet, sorbet, and frozen yogurt
Oils except canola, flaxseed, and olive oil
Pancakes and waffles not made with whole grains
Pasta and vermicelli (except for whole wheat or high-protein types)
Rice (white) and rice cakes
Snack foods (chips, pretzels)
Sugar and syrups (including honey and molasses)
White potatoes
Whole milk and whole milk products, such as butter, cheeses, and
   yogurts

Pain-Free
Recipes

WHEN CREATING THE Pain-Free Recipes, I asked my daughter, Virginia, a chef, to make sure they were simple to prepare and to use foods that are easy to find at local supermarkets. Many of my patients prepare the recipes ahead of time on the weekend and then reheat the servings during the week as they stick with the mealtime dietary requirements. Not only are the recipes delicious, but Virginia has used many anti-inflammatory foods that will help you lose weight—and pain.

In the Pain-Free Diet, we recommend using Splenda brand sweetener. Splenda, the brand name for the ingredient sucralose, is made through a patented, multistep process that starts with sugar and converts it to a no-calorie, noncarbohydrate sweetener. The result is an exceptionally stable sweetener that tastes like sugar, but without sugar's calories. After consumption, sucralose passes through the body without being broken down for energy, so it has no calories, and the body does not recognize it as a carbohydrate.

Please feel free to sweeten or otherwise season the dishes to your liking.

DRINKS

Berry Nice Smoothie

Florida Berry Granita

SALADS

Florida Orange and Spinach Salad with Sunlight Dressing

Dr. McIlwain's Salad Supreme with Olive Oil Vinaigrette Spritz

Crispy Apples, Mixed Greens, and Gorgonzola

Multibean Salad

Thai Cucumber Salad

Field, Forest, and Pond Salad

BREAKFAST

Hidden Yolk Scramble

Spanish Omelet

Cheesy Sausage Omelet

Apples and Oats

MAIN COURSES

Broiled Tuna Steak with Porcini Mushrooms and Baby Bok Choy

Sea Bass with Toasted Almonds in a Light Lemon Sauce

Indian Rocks Broiled Seafood Kabobs

So Simple Salmon

Pecan-Crusted Salmon

QUICK AND EASY

Easy Edamame (soybeans)

Broccoli Slaw

Broccolini with Garlic and Ginger

Egg and Olive Salad

Buccaneers' Sloppy Joes

Baked Apples and Cinnamon

SOUPS AND SAUCES

Apple–Butternut Squash Soup

Robust Vegetarian Chili

Dr. McIlwain's Anytime Vegetable Soup

Pesto Sauce

Thai Peanut Sauce

DRINKS

• BERRY NICE SMOOTHIE •

2 cups ice
1 cup fresh or frozen blueberries
¼ cup fresh or frozen blackberries
1 cup calcium-fortified vanilla soy milk
½ cup pineapple chunks in juice (not in syrup)
½ frozen banana
1 tablespoon Splenda
1 teaspoon lemon zest
½ teaspoons grated fresh ginger

1. In a blender, combine all ingredients and pulse until smooth.

VARIATION: Use raspberries instead of the blackberries or blueberries.

MAKES 2 SERVINGS ▪ PREPARATION TIME: 5 MINUTES

NUTRITIONAL VALUE PER SERVING: 135 calories, 8 g protein, 22 g carbohydrates, 4 g fat, and 5.5 g fiber

• FLORIDA BERRY GRANITA •

2 cups fresh or frozen blueberries, strawberries, or blackberries
½ cup Splenda
¾ teaspoon grated lime zest
1 tablespoon lime juice
2½ cups diet lemon-lime soda, chilled

1. In a blender or food processor, purée the berries until smooth, scraping the sides of the container several times. Add the Splenda, lime zest, and lime juice; process again until smooth. Pour mixture into a 1½-quart freezer container that has a cover. Pour the lemon–lime soda into the mixture, and stir. Cover the container and freeze for 12 hours. After removing from freezer, let the mixture stand for 8 minutes.

2. With an ice pick, chop the mixture into chunks. Place the chunks in a blender or food processor and pulse eight to ten times, or just until the icy mixture is smooth. Serve the granita immediately, or put it back in the freezer in its container until you are ready to consume it.

MAKES 6 SERVINGS, APPROXIMATELY 1 CUP EACH
PREPARATION TIME: 5 MINUTES; FREEZE: 12 HOURS

NUTRITIONAL VALUE PER SERVING: 30 calories, 0.3 g protein, 6.2 g carbohydrates, 0.1 g fat, and 1 g fiber

SALADS

Consider purchasing a spritz-type food-safe spray bottle. Fill the bottle with your favorite light vinaigrette dressing. Keep one bottle in your refrigerator at home and one at work, to give a light burst of flavor to your salad or steamed vegetables without overloading the food with extra calories.

• FLORIDA ORANGE AND SPINACH SALAD • WITH SUNLIGHT DRESSING

8 cups fresh spinach, washed and patted dry
1 cup mandarin oranges, canned in juice (not syrup) and drained
½ cup seedless red or green grapes, sliced in half
2 tablespoons red onion, very thinly sliced
2 tablespoons sunflower seeds

Sunlight Dressing

½ cup orange juice
Juice of 1 lime
1 tablespoon olive oil
½ teaspoon McCormick's garlic and herb mix
½ teaspoon ground cumin
Dash sea salt and fresh ground pepper

1. Arrange fresh spinach leaves on four luncheon plates. Layer on the other ingredients as follows, dividing equally among the plates: mandarin orange segments, grape halves, onion slices, and sunflower seeds.
2. Prepare the Sunlight Dressing: in a small bowl, combine the orange and lime juices; add the olive oil and spices, whisk, and pour one-quarter of the mixture over each salad. If you are serving fewer than the servings listed, store the salad in an airtight container and dressing separately for use the next day.

MAKES 4 SERVINGS ▪ PREPARATION TIME: 12 MINUTES

NUTRITIONAL VALUE PER SERVING: 95 calories, 7.5 g protein, 15 g carbohydrates, 8.5 g fat, and 4 g fiber.

• DR. MCILWAIN'S SALAD SUPREME •
WITH OLIVE OIL VINAIGRETTE SPRITZ

1 small head romaine lettuce, washed and gently dried

1 head red leaf lettuce, washed and gently dried

2 cups arugula, washed and gently dried

2 cups baby spinach, washed and gently dried

1 cucumber, halved lengthwise and chopped widthwise

1 cup broccoli florets, washed and dried

Olive Oil Vinaigrette Spritz

1 clove garlic, minced

2 teaspoons dried thyme

2 tablespoons balsamic vinegar

3 tablespoons extra-virgin olive oil

1 tablespoon lemon juice

Kosher salt and fresh ground pepper

1 small spray bottle

1. Tear the romaine and red leaf lettuce into bite-size pieces and toss in a large bowl with the arugula, baby spinach, cucumber, and broccoli florets.

2. Prepare the dressing: in a small bowl, whisk the garlic, thyme, and balsamic vinegar with a little salt and pepper. Slowly whisk in the olive oil and lemon juice, until mixed well. To serve, pour the salad dressing into a small spray bottle and spritz the salad with the vinaigrette, to coat lightly.

MAKES 6 SERVINGS ■ PREPARATION TIME: 10 MINUTES

NUTRITIONAL VALUE PER SERVING: 80 calories, 3.5 g protein, 10 g carbohydrates, 7 g fat, and 3.6 g fiber.

• CRISPY APPLES, MIXED GREENS, • AND GORGONZOLA

2 seasonal apples with skin, washed, cored, and diced

2 teaspoons lemon juice

1 (16-ounce) bag mixed baby greens

¼ cup crumbled gorgonzola cheese

Dressing

1 shallot, minced

1 clove garlic, mashed with pinch of kosher salt

½ teaspoon prepared horseradish

1 teaspoon chopped fresh thyme

2 teaspoons chopped fresh chervil

3 tablespoons apple cider vinegar

Salt and fresh ground pepper

2 tablespoons extra-virgin olive oil

1. Toss the apples with lemon juice. In a separate bowl, prepare the dressing: whisk the shallot, garlic, horseradish, herbs, and vinegar with a little salt and pepper, adding the oil in small amounts until combined.

2. Just before serving, season to taste and toss the greens and apples in a large bowl with the dressing. Top with the crumbled gorgonzola cheese.

VARIATIONS: Any type of blue cheese will work here. Also, you can use fresh, crisp pears, or an apple and a pear. Use your favorite greens. If horseradish is too spicy, substitute your favorite mustard.

MAKES 4 SERVINGS ■ PREPARATION TIME: 10 MINUTES

NUTRITIONAL VALUE PER SERVING: 125 calories, 2 g protein, 9 g carbohydrates, 12 g fat, and 2.5 g fiber

• MULTIBEAN SALAD •

½ pound fresh green beans, washed and cut into thirds
or 2 (16-ounce) cans "no salt added" beans, rinsed and drained
2 rounded teaspoons Dijon mustard
2 teaspoons Splenda
¼ cup red wine vinegar
½ teaspoon McCormick's garlic and herb mix
½ teaspoon onion powder
2 tablespoons extra-virgin olive oil
1 (16-ounce) can wax beans, rinsed and drained
1 (16-ounce) can red kidney beans, rinsed and drained
1 (4-ounce) can sliced water chestnuts, rinsed and drained
½ cup red onion, chopped
½ cup red or yellow bell pepper, chopped
½ cup celery, chopped
Salt and fresh ground pepper
Red pepper flakes (optional)

1. If using fresh green beans, steam them for 5 to 7 minutes over boiling water. Remove the beans from the steamer and cold-shock them under running water. Drain and pour into a large bowl, and set aside.
2. In a small bowl, combine the mustard, Splenda, vinegar, garlic and herbs mix, and onion powder. Whisk in the oil.
3. Add the wax beans, kidney beans, water chestnuts, bell pepper, and celery to the reserved green beans. Add salt and pepper(s) to taste, toss to coat the bean salad evenly with dressing, and serve.

MAKES 8 SERVINGS

(Store the extra servings of this salad in an airtight container
for up to 4 days in the refrigerator.)

PREPARATION TIME: 20 MINUTES

NUTRITIONAL VALUE PER SERVING: 90 calories, 3.5 g protein, 23 g carbohydrates, 7 g fat, and 5 g fiber

• THAI CUCUMBER SALAD •

½ cup seasoned rice vinegar

¼ cup water

1 tablespoon Splenda

1 tablespoon garlic, finely minced

1 tablespoon soy sauce

1 teaspoon sesame oil

½ teaspoon fresh ground pepper

2 large cucumbers, peeled and sliced

2 tablespoons toasted chopped peanuts

1. In a large bowl, stir together the rice vinegar, water, Splenda, garlic, soy sauce, sesame oil, and pepper. Add the sliced cucumbers, tossing to coat. Cover the bowl and chill for 1 hour. Add the peanuts and toss; serve. This low-calorie dish will marinate and be delicious the next day. If you have extra servings left over, store the salad in an airtight container in your refrigerator.

VARIATION: Add sliced tomatoes and thinly sliced sweet onion.

Makes 6 servings ■ Preparation time: 10 minutes

NUTRITIONAL VALUE PER SERVING: 52 calories, 1.3 g protein 5.8 g carbohydrates, 2.4 g fat, and 1 g fiber

• FIELD, FOREST, AND POND SALAD •

1¼ cup cooked bulgur (prepare according to package)
1 cup sliced water chestnuts, drained
1¼ cups shiitake mushrooms, torn
¼ cup red onion, chopped
3 scallions, chopped

1. Let the just-cooked bulgur sit with a tight-fitting lid for 30 minutes. In a large bowl, combine the bulgur with the remaining ingredients, toss, and chill until ready to serve.

VARIATION: Add diced tomatoes or any of your favorite herbs. Serve over lettuce.

Makes 4 servings ▪ Preparation time: 10 minutes to prepare, 30 minutes to steam bulgur

---

NUTRITIONAL VALUE PER SERVING: 75 calories, 2.5 g protein, 12 g carbohydrates, 0 g fat, and 3 g fiber

BREAKFAST

• HIDDEN YOLK SCRAMBLE •

1 teaspoon light olive oil

3 egg whites

1 whole egg

½ teaspoon fresh or dried parsley

1 cup fresh spinach, washed, patted dry, and chopped

Kosher salt and fresh ground pepper

½ fresh organic tomato, small, sliced into wedges

1 teaspoon balsamic vinegar

1. Heat the oil in a small nonstick skillet over medium heat. Whisk the egg whites with the whole egg and herbs. Scramble the eggs in the pan until set. Add the spinach, and salt and pepper to taste. Cook until the spinach is wilted and the eggs are done to your liking. Serve with a wedge of fresh tomato and a drizzle of balsamic vinegar.

VARIATIONS: Add some fresh basil to the tomatoes, or add chopped asparagus or canned, rinsed artichoke hearts to the scrambled eggs. You can also add chervil or tarragon to the egg mixture.

MAKES 1 SERVING ■ PREPARATION TIME: 6 MINUTES

NUTRITIONAL VALUE PER SERVING: 175 calories, 16 g protein, 2 g carbohydrates, 9 g fat, and 2 g fiber

• SPANISH OMELET •

1 teaspoon olive oil

½ cup white onion, chopped

2 cloves garlic, chopped

½ cup canned artichokes hearts (in water), rinsed, drained, and chopped

¼ cup sliced mushrooms

2 tablespoons capers (optional)

Pinch of saffron

3 egg whites beaten with 1 whole egg

2 tablespoons chopped fresh parsley

1 teaspoon dried oregano

Kosher salt and fresh ground pepper

1 ounce part-skim mozzarella cheese, shredded

1. In a small nonstick skillet, heat the oil and sauté the onions over high heat for 2 minutes. Add the garlic and lower the heat to medium-high. Cook for 1 minute. Add the chopped artichokes, mushrooms, capers, and saffron, and stir, cooking for another minute. Add the eggs and herbs. Scramble until desired doneness. Season with salt and pepper to taste. Top with the shredded cheese.

VARIATIONS: Use fresh cilantro and tomatoes instead of capers and saffron. Add fresh diced tomatoes and serve with soy sour cream.

MAKES 1 SERVING ▪ PREPARATION TIME: 10 MINUTES

NUTRITIONAL VALUE PER SERVING: 280 calories, 26 g protein, 10 g carbohydrates, 13 g fat, and 5 g fiber

• CHEESY SAUSAGE OMELET •

Nonstick cooking spray
1 whole egg
3 egg whites
Kosher salt and fresh ground pepper
1 soy sausage patty, chopped
½ ounce-shredded Gruyère cheese

1. In a small nonstick skillet, heat oil to medium temperature. In a small bowl, whisk eggs with a pinch of salt and pepper. Pour the eggs into the pan, and with a spatula push the edges toward the center, letting the uncooked eggs run to the edge and turning the pan while the eggs cook. Cook for about 2 minutes, and add the chopped soy sausage and cheese to center of the omelet. Fold or roll out onto a plate.

VARIATIONS: Consider red pepper flakes for a spicier omelet. If you prefer, try ½ ounce of 2% sharp cheddar cheese in place of gruyère cheese.

MAKES I SERVING ■ PREPARATION TIME: 6 MINUTES

NUTRITIONAL VALUE PER SERVING: 251 calories, 26 g protein, 2.7 g carbohydrates, 12 g fat, and 2 g fiber

· APPLES AND OATS ·

1 cup old-fashioned (not instant or quick) oats

1¾ cups water

½ teaspoon salt

2 seasonal apples, rinsed, cored, and diced

1 teaspoon ground cinnamon

1 tablespoon honey

1. In a medium-size saucepan, bring the oats and water to a boil and add the salt. Stir well until the oats begin to thicken, about 5 minutes. Reduce to a gentle simmer and add the cinnamon and apples; stir well. Cook uncovered for 2 to 3 minutes longer, stirring occasionally, until most of the liquid is absorbed. Add honey and serve.

VARIATIONS: Use blueberries or dried fruit instead of apples. Add 2 tablespoons of chopped walnuts.

MAKES 2 SERVINGS ■ PREPARATION TIME: 5 MINUTES
PREPARATION, 20 MINUTES COOKING TIME

NUTRITIONAL VALUE PER SERVING: 250 calories, 7 g protein, 50 g carbohydrates, 25 g fat, and 7 g fiber

MAIN COURSES

· BROILED TUNA STEAK WITH PORCINI · MUSHROOMS AND BABY BOK CHOY

4 (4-ounce) tuna steaks

1 teaspoon sea salt

1⅔ cups porcini mushrooms, sliced

3 tablespoons balsamic vinegar

1 tablespoon tamari or soy sauce

½ cup red wine

1 teaspoon Splenda

3 cloves garlic, minced

3 tablespoons olive oil

4 heads baby bok choy, halved lengthwise

1. Preheat the oven to broil.
2. Place the tuna steaks in a shallow dish and season with salt on both sides. In a separate bowl, combine the mushrooms, balsamic vinegar, tamari, red wine, sugar, garlic, and 1½ tablespoons of the olive oil. Pour the mixture over the tuna steaks and marinate in the refrigerator for 15 minutes.
3. Remove tuna steaks, leaving as much marinade in the dish as possible. Blot the steaks gently with a paper towel and brush lightly with remaining 1½ tablespoons of olive oil. Put the tuna on a grilling pan and broil in the oven on the middle rack for 3 to 4 minutes on each side to about medium doneness, or until desired doneness is achieved.
4. While the tuna steaks are cooking, in a small saucepan bring the remaining marinade to a boil and lower the heat to a simmer; cook for 2 to 3 minutes longer. Place the baby bok choy in a microwave-safe dish. Sprinkle with about 3 tablespoons of water and cover tightly. Microwave for 1 to 2 minutes, until bright green and slightly tender. Season with salt and pepper to taste. Spoon the remaining marinade on top of the fish when ready to serve, and serve with the baby bok choy.

VARIATIONS: You may use dried porcini mushrooms that have been rehydrated. One ounce of dry porcini mushrooms equals about 2 cups when rehydrated. Garnish with sliced scallions. The bok choy can also be cooked in a little simmering water, covered, in a shallow pan for 1 to 2 minutes (instead of using a microwave oven).

MAKES 4 SERVINGS ▪ PREPARATION TIME: 15 MINUTES

NUTRITIONAL VALUE PER SERVING: 225 calories, 20 g protein, 8 g carbohydrates, 12 g fat, and 2 g fiber

• SEA BASS WITH TOASTED ALMONDS • IN A LIGHT LEMON SAUCE

4 (6-ounce) Chilean sea bass fillets
Pinch of lemon zest
Kosher salt and fresh ground pepper
2 tablespoons olive oil
¼ cup dry white wine
2 teaspoons white wine vinegar
Juice of 1 lemon
1 tablespoon capers, rinsed
¼ cup slivered almonds, lightly toasted

1. Season the fillets with the lemon zest, salt, and pepper. In a large skillet, heat the oil over medium-high heat and cook the fillets for about 4 minutes on each side. Remove the fillets from the pan and keep warm. Pour the wine into the pan and stir. Add the vinegar, lemon juice, and capers, and simmer until reduced a little, about 2 minutes. Toss in the almonds. Pour the sauce over the fillets.

VARIATION: Grouper, halibut, or John Dory are good substitutes for the sea bass.

MAKES 4 SERVINGS ■ PREPARATION TIME: 15 MINUTES

NUTRITIONAL VALUE PER SERVING: 250 calories, 26 g protein, 2.5 g carbohydrates, 17 g fat, and 1.5 g fiber

• INDIAN ROCKS BROILED •
SEAFOOD KABOBS

½ cup rice wine vinegar

¼ cup water

2 teaspoons lemon juice

2 teaspoons dried chervil

1 teaspoon dried parsley

¼ teaspoon garlic powder

Pinch of salt

¾ pound sea scallops

1 pound mahimahi, cut into medium-size cubes

12 medium-size mushroom caps

2 medium-size red or green bell peppers, rinsed, seeded, and cut into large chunks

1 pint cherry tomatoes, rinsed

4 skewers

1. Mix the vinegar, water, lemon juice, chervil, parsley, garlic powder, and salt in a small bowl. Place the scallops and mahimahi in shallow baking dish, and pour the marinade on top. Let stand for 15 to 20 minutes in the refrigerator.
2. Heat the oven to broil. Line a baking dish with foil and grease lightly.
3. Drain the fish and reserve the marinade. Arrange the fish, mushrooms, peppers, scallops, and cherry tomatoes alternately on four skewers. Place the kabobs in the prepared baking dish. Broil until the fish is tender, brushing with remaining marinade, until the fish flakes with a fork, about 10 minutes. Turn the kabobs over halfway through cooking time to ensure even doneness.

MAKES 4 SERVINGS ■ PREPARATION TIME: 15 MINUTES TO PREPARE, 30 MINUTES TO MARINATE AND BROIL.

NUTRITIONAL VALUE PER SERVING: 242 calories, 38 g protein, 8g carbohydrates, 3 g fat, and 1 g fiber

• SO SIMPLE SALMON •

4 (4-ounce) fillets salmon
1 tablespoon olive oil
Kosher salt and fresh ground pepper

Sauce:

2 tablespoons stone-ground or Dijon mustard
1 teaspoon prepared horseradish
1 tablespoon Splenda
2 tablespoons lime juice, freshly squeezed
¼ cup vegetable stock

1. Preheat the oven to 400°F.
2. Make the sauce: combine the five sauce ingredients in a saucepan and bring to a simmer while stirring. Keep warm over very low heat until salmon is prepared.
3. Season the salmon fillets with a little salt and pepper on both sides. Let rest to absorb the seasoning, about 10 minutes. In a large nonstick skillet, heat the olive oil over medium-high heat. Place the salmon in the pan, fleshy side down, and cook for 3 minutes, until golden on top. Turn the salmon; if the pan is ovenproof, place it into the oven to finish cooking for another 4 minutes at 400°F. If the pan is not ovenproof, transfer the fillets to a foil baking sheet or baking dish and finish cooking in the 400°F oven for 4 minutes. Serve the sauce over the salmon.

VARIATION: Use any of your favorite coldwater fish, such as halibut, in place of salmon.

MAKES 4 SERVINGS ▪ PREPARATION TIME: 20 MINUTES

NUTRITIONAL VALUE PER SERVING: 270 calories, 21 g protein, 4 g carbohydrates, 6 g fat, and 0 g fiber

• PECAN-CRUSTED SALMON •

4 (4-ounce) salmon fillets

½ cup pecans, finely chopped

1 teaspoon Splenda

Salt

2 tablespoons orange juice

1 egg white

1. Preheat the oven to 425°F.
2. Spray a large baking sheet lightly with nonstick cooking spray, and then place the salmon fillets on the sheet with their sides touching. Bake the salmon at 425°F for 10 minutes.
3. Combine the pecans, sugar, salt, orange juice, and egg white in a small bowl. Remove the pan from the oven and pour the pecan topping evenly over the fish. Bake for an additional 10 minutes, or until cooked through.

MAKES 4 SERVINGS ■ PREPARATION TIME: 15 MINUTES TO PREPARE,
20 MINUTES TO BAKE

NUTRITIONAL VALUE PER SERVING: 275 calories, 27g protein, 5 g carbohydrates, 19 g fat, and 1 g fiber

QUICK AND EASY

• EASY EDAMAME •

1 package frozen edamame, unpeeled (look in grocer's freezer)
Sea salt

1. Microwave the frozen edamame beans in a medium-size bowl. Serve with a sprinkling of coarse sea salt. Peel and enjoy.

VARIATION: Heat a package of *peeled* edamame and sprinkle with sea salt or tamari.

MAKES 2 SERVINGS ▪ PREPARATION TIME: 5 MINUTES

NUTRITIONAL VALUE PER SERVING: 100 calories, 8 g protein, 7 g carbohydrates, 3.5 g fat, and 3 g fiber

· BROCCOLI SLAW ·

1 cup grated broccoli stems
1 cup savoy or other green cabbage, shredded
1 cup broccoli rabe or broccoli florets
½ cup celeriac (celery root, which resembles a turnip), shredded
1 tablespoon lemon juice
¼ cup soy sour cream
3 tablespoons rice vinegar
Kosher salt and fresh ground pepper

1. Place all the shredded vegetables in a large bowl. In a small bowl, combine the lemon juice, soy sour cream, and vinegar, and stir until mixed well. Season with salt and pepper. Mix the sour cream dressing with the vegetables.

VARIATIONS: Add shredded carrots, green onions, or julienned bell peppers. Add 1 tablespoon of Splenda to the dressing for a sweeter slaw.

MAKES 4 SERVINGS ■ PREPARATION TIME: 10 MINUTES

NUTRITIONAL VALUE PER SERVING: 50 calories, 0.5 g protein, 0.8 g carbohydrates, 1 g fat, and 1 g fiber

· BROCCOLINI WITH GARLIC AND GINGER ·

2 tablespoons olive oil
1 bunch broccolini (a cross between broccoli and Chinese kale),
washed and ends trimmed
1 clove garlic, minced
1 tablespoon ginger, minced
4 tablespoons vegetable stock or water
Kosher salt and fresh ground pepper

1. In a medium-size skillet, heat the oil over medium heat. Sauté the broccolini, garlic, and ginger for 2 minutes. Add the stock and cover; steam for 1 or 2 minutes. Season with salt and pepper to taste.

VARIATIONS: Add crushed red pepper flakes or julienned red peppers.

Makes 4 servings ■ Preparation time: 6 minutes

NUTRITIONAL VALUE PER SERVING: 80 calories, 4 g protein, 10 g carbohydrates, 3.5 g fat, and 3.5 g fiber

• EGG AND OLIVE SALAD •

4 eggs

1 cup egg substitute

3 tablespoons light mayonnaise

4 tablespoons sliced green olives

2 tablespoons chopped scallions or sweet onions

Salt and fresh ground pepper

1. In a medium-size saucepan, cover the eggs with cold water and bring to a rolling boil over high heat. Reduce the heat to a medium-low and boil for an additional 12 minutes. Remove the eggs from the pan and plunge immediately into a bowl of ice water.

2. Spray a skillet with a nonstick cooking spray and heat; pour 1 cup egg substitute into the hot pan and slowly scramble. Transfer the scrambled egg substitute to a plate and let cool.

3. Carefully remove shells from the hard-boiled eggs. Put the eggs in a medium-size bowl and chop well. Add scrambled egg substitute and mix. Stir in the mayonnaise, olives, and scallions. Add salt and pepper to taste, and serve.

VARIATION: Add chopped celery for crunch.

MAKES 4 SERVINGS ■ PREPARATION TIME: 5 MINUTES PREPARATION, 20 MINUTES TO COOK AND COOL EGGS

NUTRITIONAL VALUE PER SERVING: 150 calories, 13.2 g protein, 2.45 g carbohydrates, 10.2 g fat, and 1 g fiber

• BUCCANEERS' SLOPPY JOES •

2 tablespoons olive oil

1 onion, diced

2 medium-size green bell peppers, rinsed, seeded, and diced

12 ounces soy burger crumbles (look in grocer's freezer)

1 (16-ounce) can tomato sauce

1 tablespoon chile powder

1 teaspoon garlic powder

1 teaspoon mustard powder

½ teaspoon oregano

2 tablespoons Splenda brown sugar

1. In a large skillet, sauté the onion and green pepper in the olive oil and stir, cooking over medium heat for several minutes. Add the soy crumbles and continue to cook, stirring occasionally to keep the textured vegetable protein from burning. Add the tomato sauce, spices, and Splenda, and stir. Simmer for 10 to 15 minutes over medium to medium-low heat, stirring until well combined. Serve on a whole wheat bun.

MAKES 4 SERVINGS ■ PREPARATION TIME: 20 MINUTES

NUTRITIONAL VALUE PER SERVING: 225 calories, 18g protein, 21 g carbohydrates, 10 g fat, and 6.5 g fiber.

• BAKED APPLES AND CINNAMON •

8 rome apples, rinsed, cored, and sliced in ½-inch slices
1 (12-ounce) can diet cream soda or root beer
2 tablespoons ground cinnamon
2 tablespoons Splenda brown sugar mix

1. Preheat the oven to 350°F.
2. Arrange the apple slices in a baking dish. Pour the soda over the apples and bake uncovered at 350°F for 30 minutes. Combine the cinnamon and Splenda, and sprinkle over the apples, stirring into the baked fruit. Serve warm, cold, or partially frozen.

VARIATION: Top with 1 tablespoon chopped walnuts or light Cool Whip.

MAKES 8 SERVINGS ■ PREPARATION TIME: 5 MINUTES TO PREPARE,
30 MINUTES BAKING TIME

NUTRITIONAL VALUE PER SERVING: 60 calories, 0.4 g protein, 16 g carbohydrates, 0 g fat, and 1.7 g fiber

SOUPS AND SAUCES

• APPLE–BUTTERNUT SQUASH SOUP •

2 medium-size butternut squash

1 large apple, peeled, cored, and diced

1 tablespoon olive oil

1 large onion, diced

2 cups water

¼ teaspoon fresh ground nutmeg

¼ teaspoon dried oregano

½ teaspoon garlic powder

1 teaspoon curry powder

1 cup apple juice

1 cup soy milk

Scallions, chopped, for garnish (optional)

Dollop of light or soy sour cream, for garnish (optional)

1. Preheat the oven to 350°F. Cut the butternut squash in half lengthwise and scoop out the flesh, discarding the seeds and strings. Bake squash skinside down at 350°F on a non-stick baking sheet (or spray with non-stick cooking spray) for 40 minutes.

2. Sauté onion in the olive oil in a large saucepan over medium heat. Cook for several minutes, and then add squash and diced apple. Cook for several more minutes. Add the water and seasonings, and bring to a boil. Cover the pot and simmer, stirring occasionally, for 10 minutes.

3. Transfer the mixture to a blender or food processor, and pulse until creamy. Pour back into the saucepan. Add the apple juice and soy milk, and simmer an additional 5 to 10 minutes. Add salt and pepper to taste, and garnish with scallions or a dollop of light or soy sour cream.

MAKES 4 SERVINGS ▪ PREPARATION TIME: 30 MINUTES TO PREPARE
AND COOK SOUP; 40 MINUTES BAKING TIME

NUTRITIONAL VALUE PER SERVING: 210 calories, 6 g protein, 36 g carbohydrates, 4 g fat, and 4 g fiber

• ROBUST VEGETARIAN CHILI •

3 teaspoons olive oil

1 large onion, chopped

1 large green bell pepper, rinsed, seeded, and chopped

1 clove garlic, minced

12 ounces soy burger crumbles (look in grocer's freezer)

2 (15-ounce) cans seasoned chili beans

1 (15-ounce) can tomato sauce

2 cups hot water

1 cup carrots, rinsed, trimmed, and finely chopped

1 tablespoon Splenda

1. In a small skillet, sauté the onion, green pepper, and garlic in 1 teaspoon of the olive oil over medium heat until soft (use nonstick cooking spray if needed to keep it from sticking). In a large saucepan, sauté the soy burger crumbles in the remaining 2 teaspoons of oil over medium heat until cooked through, 5 to 10 minutes. Add the beans, tomato sauce, water, carrots, and sugar to the saucepan. Bring to a boil. Simmer for 30 minutes. Add more water if the chili is too thick.

VARIATIONS: Serve with scallions and a dollop of low-fat or soy sour cream. Top with jalapeños.

MAKES 4 SERVINGS ▪ PREPARATION TIME: 15 MINUTES TO PREPARE,
30 MINUTES TO SIMMER

NUTRITIONAL VALUE PER SERVING: 250 calories, 23 g protein, 17 g carbohydrates, 7 g fat, and 4.5 g fiber.

• DR. MCILWAIN'S •
ANYTIME VEGETABLE SOUP

Nonstick cooking spray

1 large sweet onion, chopped

4 red or yellow bell peppers, rinsed and chopped

2 cups small button mushrooms, rinsed

1 small head of cabbage, rinsed, cored, and thinly sliced

2 cans petite tomatoes, chopped; or, to reduce sodium,

4 large fresh tomatoes, chopped

4 carrots, rinsed and sliced

1 bunch celery, rinsed and thinly sliced

6 cups low-sodium vegetable broth

1 (48-ounce) can low-sodium V8 juice or tomato juice

1 teaspoon McCormick's garlic and herb mix

1 tablespoon onion powder

½ teaspoon red pepper flakes (optional)

1 teaspoon sweet basil

1 tablespoon Splenda

2 bay leaves

Kosher salt and fresh ground pepper

1. Spray a large saucepan with nonstick cooking spray, and sauté the onion, peppers, and mushrooms for about 5 minutes. Add the cabbage and sauté about 5 minutes longer to combine flavors. Add the remaining ingredients and cook for 1 hour, stirring occasionally. You can adjust the thickness by adding more water as it cooks (do not let it get too thick). Remove bay leaves before serving. This is a delicious soup that has virtually zero calories, but it is nutritious and will fill you up when you need a snack between meals. Store in the refrigerator in an airtight container for up to 4 days.

VARIATION: Dr. McIlwain's favorite soup is delicious served cold like gazpacho.

MAKES 8 SERVINGS ■ PREPARATION TIME: 15 MINUTES TO PREPARE,
I HOUR TO SIMMER.

• PESTO SAUCE •

2 large cloves garlic
2 cups packed fresh basil leaves
3 tablespoons pine nuts
2 tablespoons lemon juice
4 tablespoons fresh parmesan cheese
⅓ cup olive oil

1. Blend all the ingredients in a blender or food processor. Add additional lemon juice to taste for a smoother consistency.
2. Serve over Barilla PLUS high-protein pasta. This sauce stores well in an airtight container in the refrigerator for several days.

MAKES 6 SERVINGS ▪ PREPARATION TIME: 5 MINUTES TO PREPARE

NUTRITIONAL VALUE PER SERVING: 150 calories, 2 g protein, 2 g carbohydrates, 14 g fat, and 1.5 g fiber.

• THAI PEANUT SAUCE •

1 tablespoon canola oil

1 clove garlic, minced

¼ cup onion, finely chopped

3 tablespoons peanut butter

5 tablespoons water

2 teaspoons rice vinegar

1 tablespoon soy sauce

1 tablespoon lemon juice

1 teaspoon honey

½ teaspoon garlic powder

½ teaspoon onion powder

¼ teaspoon cayenne pepper

1. Heat the oil in a small saucepan. Sauté the onion and garlic over medium heat for 3 to 4 minutes, until translucent. Add the peanut butter and stir until combined. Add the rest of the ingredients, and stir. Simmer for several minutes, until thick and creamy. For a smoother sauce, blend the mixture in a food processor or blender. You may wish to add more water for a thinner sauce.

2. Serve on any combination of steamed vegetables (broccoli, carrots, red and green peppers, yellow squash, onion, cauliflower, and mushrooms).

MAKES 4 SERVINGS ■ PREPARATION TIME: 5 MINUTES TO PREPARE

NUTRITIONAL VALUE PER SERVING: 110 calories, 3.5 g protein, 4 g carbohydrates, 10 g fat, and 0.5 g fiber

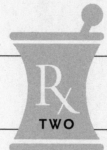

TWO

Exercise
Your Pain
Away

Exercise
Your Pain Away

The most effective way to stop pain is to **keep your body active**—*daily*—*moving in full range of motion and keeping your cardiovascular system in optimal health.*

URSULA, A FORMER college basketball player, knows all about living with pain, specifically the pain of osteoarthritis. When I first met her, she told me, "At forty-one, I am living proof that you don't have to be old to feel wear and tear on your joints. Not only do my knees hurt when I get out of bed each morning, but after doing yard work or even standing for a short period of time, I have to soak in our Jacuzzi and take pain medication for relief."

Ursula's story is one you may relate to: she was a star athlete as a teenager and young adult, had a sedentary career as a software engineer, experienced a weight gain of 40 pounds since having two children, and now her knees hurt "all day, every day." While she knows that exercise is vital for good health, Ursula could not remember the last time she really tried to get back in shape and lamented, "When I exercise, my knees hurt so badly, I immediately stop. Why should I inflict more pain than I have to?"

I explained to Ursula how her weight and sedentary lifestyle contributed to the arthritic knee pain, and suggested that she consider starting the Pain-Free Diet and exercise plan to lose weight and strengthen the muscles that support the knees. Desperate for relief, Ursula started the Pain-Free Diet last year. In 21 days, she lost 6 pounds and was riding a stationary bike for more than 30 minutes each day. Ursula felt such relief from her knee pain and stiffness that she urged her husband and mother to join her on the program.

After following the program for six months, Ursula lost a total of 21 pounds and dropped 4 inches from her waistline. She felt in control of her life for the first time in years. Her husband, Bill, who had suffered back pain from a ruptured disc, lost 36 pounds on the program and 3 inches from his waist. And her mother, Ellen, who had back pain from a fractured vertebra, lost 18 pounds and 2 inches from her waist. Today, Ursula, Bill, and Ellen are thrilled that they can be as active as they want to be. They enjoy outdoor activities at their lake cottage on weekends and look forward to living pain free for many years to come.

Jim's Lower Back Pain

Likewise, Jim's experience is another you might be familiar with. This fifty-six-year-old project manager was thin, muscular, and extremely active during young adulthood, playing on the company softball team and coaching his kids' baseball and swim teams. In fact, Jim used to drink high-fat milkshakes between meals to try to gain weight . . . until he turned forty. At that time, he noticed that he was getting "belly fat." While he had only gained about 15 pounds, the weight was all in his waistline, which went from 33 to 36 inches over a period of a few years.

When I saw Jim, he complained of overall aches and pains, particularly after standing or sitting at his computer for a period of time. Looking at Jim's lab results, I noticed that his C-reactive protein level was elevated. His LDL cholesterol, triglycerides, and blood pressure were all higher since his last visit. While Jim was not in a danger zone, the increases were significant warning signs that he needed to lose weight and start exercising.

I told Jim about the diet and explained how daily exercise works to decrease pro-inflammatory markers, as well as reduce his cholesterol and blood pressure. As with Ursula, it was not easy to convince him to exercise. But about two weeks later, Jim called the clinic for more information. He had spent several hours bending over, trying to fix broken sprinklers. When he finally stood up, he felt excruciating pain in his lower back. He needed relief for his pain and was willing to try anything.

Jim lost 9 pounds in 3 weeks when he followed Rx #1 of Pain-Free Diet. And just as Ursula and her family experienced, he felt good pain relief and was able to start exercising daily, which strengthened his muscles and increased his flexibility. Within three months, Jim had lost 16 pounds and his waist measurement dropped to 34 inches. His C-reactive protein level also dropped—by a startling 50 percent—and his blood pressure was back in a safe range.

Ursula and Jim are just two patients among many who have experienced tremendous results with the Pain-Free Diet and today are able to be extremely active, including daily exercise, without pain or limitations. But so many people, particularly baby boomers, are still living with loss of muscle mass, decreased bone density, muscle and tendon flexibility and joints that are stiff and less able to respond to impact. The longer you are inactive and sedentary, the more your muscles lose strength and work less efficiently. Inactivity also increases fatigue, achiness, and an inability to handle stress, as well as the risk of high blood pressure, high cholesterol, and type 2 diabetes.

When you combine a sedentary lifestyle with aging, the result is often chronic pain. Sitting on the sidelines for months at a time results in significant deficits in muscle and bone strength and flexibility and can increase pro-inflammatory markers in the body.

HOW EXERCISE REDUCES WAIST SIZE, INFLAMMATION, AND PAIN

For the past two decades, many doctors have had a simple solution for chronic pain: they wrote prescriptions for pain medications. While I believe in the relief some medications can bring to suffering, medications play only a partial role in alleviating long-term pain. The most effective way to stop pain is to *keep your body functioning*—daily—in full range of motion and keep your cardiovascular system in optimal health.

Many popular weight-loss programs claim to reduce markers of inflammation simply by diet alone, but scientific studies fail to substantiate this outcome. A revealing study from Duke University evaluated the effects of varying amounts and intensities of exercise in sedentary overweight men and women. Duke researchers found that in study participants who did not exercise, visceral fat rapidly accumulated deep in the subjects' abdomens and their waist size increased. In contrast, the participants who exercised using a treadmill, elliptical trainer, or stationary bicycle had significant declines in abdominal fat. Over time, the participants who did not exercise experienced an 8.6 percent increase in abdominal fat over eight months. The exercising participants had an 8.1 percent decrease in abdominal fat.

Studies such as the one from Duke are beginning to unravel the intimate relationship between exercise and inflammation. Researchers have observed that aerobic or conditioning exercise significantly reduces pro-inflammatory markers in the body. In one study, moderate exercisers were found to be 15 percent less likely than sedentary individuals to have elevated C-reactive protein levels. In addition, those volunteers who exercised vigorously were 47 percent less likely to have a high C-reactive protein level than their sedentary peers.

In another revealing study, obese men with metabolic syndrome (page 8), were placed on a high-fiber, low-fat diet with daily *aerobic exercise* in a three-week residential program. After three weeks on the regimen, the study participants experienced significant reductions in body mass index, fasting glucose and insulin, and inflammatory markers. In fact, a startling 9 of the 15 men were no longer positive for metabolic syndrome! Researchers concluded that intensive lifestyle modification of a low-fat, high fiber diet combined with conditioning exercise led to a better balance between inflammatory and anti-inflammatory responses.

As you start the exercise step, continue to rate your pain each week, using the 10-point questionnaire on pages 26 to 27, and write down your Pain Quotient. Compare the weekly Pain Quotients to see if your pain is decreasing (or increasing) over time. As stated, if your Pain Quotient is increasing, talk to your doctor to see if a change in medication is necessary or if you need to be evaluated for another problem that may be causing your pain. It's also important to weigh yourself and to measure your hips and waist each week, as you keep tabs on your BMI and hip-waist ratio.

More Exercise Perks

EXERCISE SLOWS DOWN the heart-racing adrenaline associated with stress, and boosts levels of endorphins (proteins that reduce feelings of pain and induce euphoria). Exercise also helps to relieve low-grade depression and aids in achieving quality, restful sleep.

Banish Belly Fat!

In the forty patients who followed the Pain-Free Diet, after six months following the four prescriptions, almost all the participants had lost 3 to 6 inches from their respective waistlines. One woman, Nancy, age 47, suffered with the deep muscle pain of fibromyalgia syndrome and had not exercised for almost a decade until she committed to this study. Nancy went from a 38-inch waist to 33 inches. Her C-reactive protein level dropped about 40 percent, too. Not only did this mother of three dramatically lower her risk of chronic illness, her pain assessment score dropped to a very tolerable 2 out of 10 on most days, with less medication.

Another patient, fifty-four-year-old Raymond, who had *ankylosing spondilitis*, a type of arthritis that causes tremendous pain and stiffness in the back, went from a 40-inch waist to 35 inches during the six-month trial. Raymond's BMI decreased 6 percent, and his C-reactive protein level dropped 35 percent. Raymond said that his back pain was greatly improved on most days.

Not only are a large waist and belly fat critical measurements that indicate the presence of chronic inflammation, a large waist can increase shoulder, neck, and back pain, particularly in women. In one Japanese study, researchers found that the waist-to-hip ratio was higher in women with generalized back pain, meaning that these women were more likely than others in the study to have excess abdominal fat. They also, on average, had less muscle in their back and legs than other study participants. Another similar study found that women who have large waists have a significantly increased likelihood of low back pain.

The *American Journal of Public Health* published revealing findings that substantiate these studies: large waist circumferences and high BMI scores are associated with impaired quality of life and disability that hinder basic activities of daily living. But you don't need a study to tell you that a large abdomen results in strain and overstretching of ligaments and muscles, increased compression on joints and disks. If you have a large belly, your back will try to support the extra weight out in front by swaying backward, causing excess strain on the lower back muscles. Excess weight and muscle imbalance increase stress on joints and soft tissues.

In the Long Run, Exercise Will Make Your Pain Better, Not Worse

Many of my patients initially balk at the word *exercise*. Isabella, age 54, who later became an avid supporter of this pain-free program, expressed her thoughts honestly when she said, "Dr. McIlwain, even hearing you mention the word *exercise* makes me feel tired and sore." But when I explain that daily activities such as gardening, grocery shopping, mowing the lawn, and housekeeping are all considered exercise and are part of the Pain-Free lifestyle approach, patients like Isabella become more accepting.

There comes a time when each of us has to make some dramatic changes in our exercise routine. For most people over age forty this means moving from the couch (or more likely the computer chair) onto a treadmill or stationary bike. In my practice, I've found that many patients who suffer with ongoing pain are sedentary out of fear of experiencing more pain. I also see many semifit and unfit weekend warriors who suffer repeatedly with sports injuries and may need to accept their age and physical condition. They should reconsider their extreme sports regimen, instead selecting activities that are conditioning and strengthening but that also reduce the chance of injury.

I have demonstrated that almost anyone—no matter what the person's age or weight—can start a daily exercise and activity program. Of course, if you have been sedentary for a long period of time, you may initially have aches and pains and stiffness when you start to exercise. These are temporary feelings that subside once you begin to get in shape and exercise regularly. To avoid this problem, start your exercise program slowly, and progress over time while focusing on building muscle strength and flexibility and increasing range of motion in the joints. When you combine the Pain-Free Diet with conditioning exercise, you will boost weight loss and decrease inflammation.

It's Never Too Late to Start Moving Again

No matter what your pain problem, it is important to find activities that will keep you trim and strengthen your cardiovascular system, muscles, and bones. In this step, I want to redefine exercise to include enjoyable activities. When you obtain pleasure from an activity or exercise, the chances are greater that you will stick with the plan. I will discuss how conditioning exercise can be easily done throughout your day and how functional fitness exercises can help to strengthen muscles and keep your joints lubricated and moving in a full range of motion. I will also explain some functional movements that focus on training your body to control and balance its own weight. These exercises will help you stay active throughout the day so you can take care of activities of daily living, along with balancing other responsibilities such as a household, career, and family.

THE PAIN-FREE FUNCTIONAL
FITNESS EXERCISES

While daily exercise and activity are a critical part of this step in the Pain-Free program, I do not expect you to start training for marathons. Rather, try to focus on *functional fitness exercises* that strengthen and stabilize your body so you can easily perform your daily activities. My patients who do these exercises are able to stay extremely active well into retirement years, doing the recreational sports and activities they enjoy, including travel. They also find it's easier to maintain a normal weight because they are able to be active.

The three categories of functional fitness exercises in the Pain-Free program, include the following:

1. **Range of Motion**—moving your joints while strengthening your muscles using light one-pound weights
2. **Stretching**—moving your body gently while stabilizing and balancing your weight
3. **Conditioning**—with exercise and activities

Find the Exercise That's Best for Your Pain

TYPE OF PAIN AND/ OR PAINFUL CONDITIONS	BEST PAIN-FREE EXERCISE CHOICE
Ankle Pain	Range of motion exercises (page 152), swimming, indoor stationary bicycling with low resistance, strengthening legs
Back pain	Range-of-motion exercises, strengthening exercises, resistance with light weights, swimming, crunches to strengthen abdominal muscles
Carpal tunnel syndrome	Walking, water aerobics, stretching, yoga, tai chi, range-of-motion exercises (avoid repetitive exercises for the wrist)
Fibromyalgia syndrome	Stretching, range-of-motion exercises, strengthening, walking, swimming, stationary bicycling, water exercises in a heated pool

Hip pain	Indoor stationary bicycling with low resistance, range-of-motion exercises, and strengthening back and legs
Knee pain	Indoor stationary bicycling to strengthen the muscles of the thigh and support the knee; strengthening quadriceps, hamstrings, back muscles
Neck pain	Stretching, range-of-motion exercises, walking, yoga, shoulder and back exercises, (talk to your doctor or physical therapist for specific exercises)
Osteoarthritis	Swimming, water exercises, yoga, tai chi, Pilates, stretching and strengthening, (talk to your doctor or physical therapist for specific exercises)
Osteoporosis	Weight-bearing exercise (walking, jogging, running, aerobics, stair climbing, dancing, tennis), specific back exercises after instruction by your doctor or physical therapist
Rheumatoid and other inflammatory types of arthritis	Stretching, range-of-motion exercises, strengthening. (Talk to your doctor or physical therapist for specific exercises)
Shoulder pain	Water aerobics, range-of-motion exercises, strengthening, swimming
Tennis elbow	Stretching specifically for tennis elbow (talk to your doctor or physical therapist), yoga, tai chi, range-of-motion exercises

1. Strengthening Your Muscles and Joints with Range-of-Motion Exercises

How often: Start gradually; work toward a goal of 20 repetitions of each exercise, twice daily

Range-of-motion exercises are the first category of exercises in the Pain-Free program. You can do these simple exercises at home or at work, and they are crucial to keeping your joints functioning properly and your muscles strong and pliable. These exercises also help strengthen and stabilize the muscles of your back, shoulders, and legs—important for preventing falls.

As you do these twice daily, you will notice that your daily activities become easier. Because your body is more functional, it becomes easier to bend, lift, push, and pull throughout your day.

As part of your Pain-Free program, do the following exercises twice daily after a warm shower, bath, or Jacuzzi soak. Start with only 1 or 2 repetitions of each exercise, then as you feel comfortable at this level, gradually increase as you can up to 5, then 10, with a goal of 20 repetitions in the morning and again at night. If you experience too much pain or stiffness, cut back to half as many exercises. You can try doing the exercises in your warm shower, tub, or Jacuzzi for extra pain relief. If you have pain after exercising, it usually means that you did too much, so lower by half or more if needed until you feel less pain. Then you can start back on your program and gradually increase toward the goal.

Shoulders

These exercises will help you move your shoulder in a full range of motion. Start slowly and don't force movement. Apply shower or moist heat pad to the shoulders if you find the exercises painful. You will gradually build strength and flexibility if you perform these exercises daily.

- While standing or sitting, clasp your hands behind your head. Pull your elbows together until they are as close as possible in front of your chin. Separate your elbows to the side as much as possible. Repeat, gradually increasing to 5, then 10, then up to 20 repetitions.
- Make large arm circles. Starting with your arms at your sides, bring them all the way up toward the ceiling and then as far behind your body as comfortable, in a huge circle. Repeat.
- While standing or sitting, roll shoulders in a forward circle; raise shoulders toward the ears in a shrugging motion. Roll shoulders back and push chest out as in a military stance. Lower the shoulders and bring the shoulders forward. Think of it as a simple shoulder roll in a circle. Now reverse the process, rolling your shoulder girdle in a backward circle.

Hips

These stretching exercises will help increase range of motion in your hips and knees, and keep you flexible. Soaking in a Jacuzzi or warm bath before and after performing the exercises will help to keep you flexible and decrease pain and stiffness.

- Lie on your back with your knees bent, feet on the floor and arms down along your sides. Bend each knee to your chest, one at a time. If you need to, put your hands under a knee and help it bend to your chest. Repeat this, alternating knees. Do 5, then 10, then 20 repetitions twice daily, if possible (see figure 2.1).
- Now bring both knees to your chest at the same time. Hold for 6 seconds. Gently rock from side to side while holding your knees. Repeat this exercise, increasing gradually to 5, then 10, then 20 repetitions two or three times a day, if possible.
- Lying on your back, move your feet and legs in the air as if you were riding a bicycle. Count to 6, and relax. Repeat, then gradually increase to 5 and then 10 repetitions once or twice daily, if tolerated.

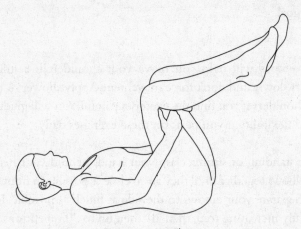

Figure 2.1—Hip Flexion

Back

These exercises will help to stretch and strengthen your back muscles and increase flexibility in your back, hips, and knees.

- Lie on your back on the floor or in bed, and bend your hips and knees. Now, raise your hips and buttocks 4 to 6 inches off the surface, forcing the small of your back out flat; and tighten your buttock and hip muscles to maintain this position. Hold this position for a count of 6 seconds. Now, relax and lower your hips and buttocks to rest again on the surface. Repeat this exercise (see figure 2.2).

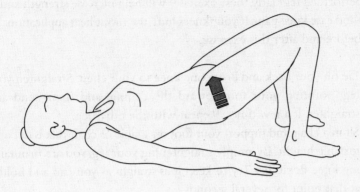

Figure 2.2—Bridging

■ The position for this exercise is a crawling position with your hands placed directly under your shoulders. Take a deep breath and arch your back like a camel's or as a frightened cat looks, lowering your head. Hold that position while you count 6 seconds out loud. Now, exhale and straighten your back slowly, raising your head. Start this exercise slowly, with 1 or 2 repetitions. Increase to 5 and then 10 repetitions, if possible (see figure 2.3).

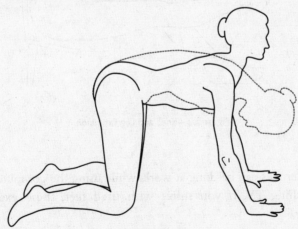

Figure 2.3—Bridging

Knees

If performed regularly, these exercises will help increase strength and flexibility and ease knee pain. If your knees hurt, use moist heat applications (page 153) before and after this exercise.

- Lie on your back and bring one knee to your chest. Straighten your leg, pointing your foot toward the ceiling, and then bend and straighten it a few times. Repeat with the other leg.
- Sit in a chair and support your foot on a table or chair that is of comfortable height. By simply straightening your leg, you are maintaining knee flexibility. Try to keep it as straight as you can and hold it at that point for several seconds.
- While sitting with one foot on a table or chair, as above, try raising your toes up so the back of your leg is stretched. Tighten your kneecap by pushing your knee down a little, and hold the contraction for 6 seconds, relax, and repeat. Begin gradually and work up to 12 repetitions at one time. Repeat this 2 or 3 times a day. You can do this exercise at work or while watching TV at night (see figure 2.4).

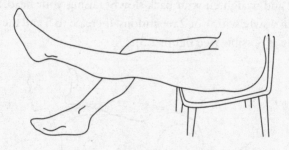

Figure 2.4—Knee and Leg Extension

Ankles

These exercises can be done at work, while using the computer, or even while watching TV. If you suffer with tired feet, these exercises are invigorating.

- While sitting in a comfortable chair, raise your toes as high as you can while keeping your heel on the floor. Then keep your toes down, while raising your heel as high as possible (see figure 2.5).

- Now, rotate the ankle, curling your toes up and down, and around in a circle.

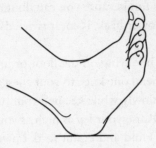

Figure 2.5—Foot Exercise

Wrists

Whether you work at a computer or use it for pleasure, it's important to stop every 30 minutes and exercise your fingers and wrists.

- Make circles with your wrists, rotating hands in both directions.

Other Exercises

Chair Lift: Sit in a straightback chair. Slowly stand up and then sit back down, using the large muscles of the leg. If you need to rely on your arms initially, that's fine. But as you progress, depend more on your leg muscles. Mastering this exercise will increase your confidence in daily activities.

Cheek to Cheek: This is a convenient exercise because you can do it anywhere, anytime, and in practically any position. It strengthens the buttock muscles that help support your back and legs. When sitting, you will actually rise up out of the chair because of the contraction of the muscle groups in your buttocks.

Press your buttocks together and hold for a 6-second count. Relax and repeat. Gradually increase up to 5, then 10, then 20 repetitions. Repeat two times daily.

Do this exercise frequently during the day, for a gentle lower body stretch.

Wall Push: This exercise is good for your back because it encourages the body extension positions.

Stand spread-eagled with your back against a solid wall. Now arch your back inward slowly. Gradually increase repetitions from 1 to 5 or more. This exercise is fun because you can do it any time you feel you feel tension in your lower back. Repeat twice daily.

Straight Leg Raise: While lying on the floor or in bed, bend your knee slightly as shown, or bend one knee to your chest if you have back pain. Raise your other leg slowly while keeping your back firmly on the surface (see figure 2.6). Raise your leg as high as you can, but stop if your back begins to arch. Hold and count to 6. Lower your leg, and then repeat with the opposite leg. Repeat for both legs, gradually increasing to 5, then 10, then 20 repetitions, twice daily. If you have severe pain with this or any exercise, stop immediately and talk to your doctor.

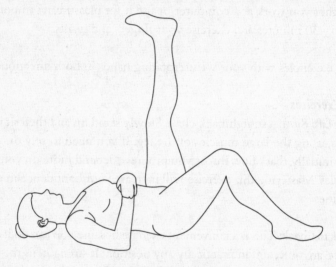

Figure 2.6—Straight Leg Raise

Add Light Weights

As you become accustomed to the range-of-motion exercises and can do 20 repetitions of each exercise twice daily, add 1- or 2-pound weights that strap onto your ankle or wrist. You can purchase the light weights from a sporting goods store. Adding the weights to the exercises will help to prevent or delay muscle atrophy, which starts to occur around middle age. I have seen that an increase in muscle strength is accompanied by a dramatic reduction in pain and disability for most of my patients, and an increase in their flexibility and body stabilization.

With each decade after age fifty, we lose about 6 percent of our muscle mass. This can cause a loss of 10 to 15 percent of strength. The problem is that losing muscle makes you physically weaker and less functional, making it more difficult to carry in groceries or walk up a flight of stairs. Losing muscle also makes it more difficult to maintain a normal weight or lose weight, because muscle is metabolically active tissue and burns more calories than fat. (Fat only burns 2 to 3 calories per pound; muscle burns 50 calories per pound.) The more muscle mass you have, the more calories your body will burn each day. This is why men can typically lose weight more quickly, while it takes most women a few weeks to drop pounds.

When you begin using the light weights with the range-of-motion exercises, go slow. Once you can easily perform the range-of-motion exercises, try the following exercises with the light weights attached to the ankle and wrist:

Upper Body Strengthening

- Standing or sitting with the light weight strapped around your wrist, raise your arm upward toward your head and then back to the side of your body. Repeat once, then twice; gradually increase up to 10 times, twice daily.
- Do arm circles with the 1-pound weight strapped around your wrist. Start with a small circle, and then gradually increase the size of the circle. Repeat once, then twice; gradually increase up to 10 times twice daily, if you can do this without pain.

Lower Body Strengthening

- Lying on your back with the 1-pound weight strapped just above your ankle, slide one leg out to the side and back to the middle. Now, do this with the other legs. Repeat once, then twice; gradually increase up to 10 times twice daily.
- Sitting in a chair, with the weight strapped at your ankle, straighten out your knee and lower it back down to the floor. Be sure to go only as far as is comfortable, and use only 1-pound weights for this resistance exercise. Repeat once, then twice, and then gradually increase up to 5 or 10 times twice daily, if you can do so without pain.

Maura's Pain-Free Back

I treated Maura, age 53, for moderate low back pain for three years. This woman wasn't more than 10 pounds above a normal weight. Still, she started the Pain-Free Diet for the inflammatory benefit and found that she did alleviate much of her pain. Yet when she started the Pain-Free exercises, she was overly enthusiastic and overdid it the first week, resulting in stiff muscles and more back pain. I explained to Maura the importance of starting exercise again, but this time she had to start slowly and progress gradually. Also, I recommended that she take a warm shower for 5 minutes each morning to help ease her back pain and stiffness, and then do some of the exercises in the shower while the warm water continued to pour on her neck and lower back. (The other exercises given on pages 154 to 155 should be done after showering, because of the space they require.)

Maura found that this easy morning shower-exercise regimen only took a few minutes; and, the longer she stayed with this program, the less pain and stiffness she felt and the easier it was to be active throughout the day. She soon realized that the payback in improved pain, stiffness, and function was well worth the time she spent each morning.

Over time, Maura was able to move into a comprehensive Pain-Free exercise program each day with swimming, water exercises, crunches to strengthen her abdominal muscles (most necessary for a pain-free back), short walks, range-of-motion exercises and stretching, and housework, among other activities. You can review her weekly exercise chart as you begin to formulate your own Pain-Free exercise plan. Using a calendar, write in your exercise times for the entire week. Fill in the time of day, type of exercise, and time allotment, so you have a good idea of the various types of exercise you will perform. I find that when patients don't plan ahead for exercise, they tend to let other commitments or interruptions stop them from being active. To live pain free, you must make a daily commitment to move around more with exercise and activities.

Maura's Pain-Free Exercise Calendar for Back Pain

DAY OF THE WEEK	TIME OF DAY	TYPE OF EXERCISE	DURATION OF EXERCISE
Monday	6:45 AM	Warm shower/range-of-motion exercises	10 minutes
	7:00 AM	Early morning swim	15 minutes
	Noon	Vacuuming and windows (housecleaning)	10 minutes
	6:00 PM	Warm shower/range-of-motion exercises	10 minutes
Tuesday	7:00 AM	Warm shower/range-of-motion exercises	10 minutes
	2:00 PM	Aquatics class at Y	20 minutes
	2:30 PM	Resistance with light weights/crunches	15 minutes
Wednesday	7:00 AM	Warm shower/range-of-motion exercises/ crunches	15 minutes
	5:00 PM	Water exercise with kickboard (flotation)	30 minutes
Thursday	7:00 AM	Warm shower/range-of-motion exercises	15 minutes
	5:00 PM	Swimming	15 minutes
Friday	7:00 AM	Swimming	20 minutes
	5:00 PM	Walking dog	10 minutes
	5:15 PM	Stretches, crunches, range-of-motion exercises	10 minutes
Saturday	7:00 AM	Housecleaning (heavy cleaning, dusting, vacuuming)	60 minutes
	5:00 PM	Stretches, crunches	10 minutes
Sunday	Noon	Swimming	15 minutes
	12:30 PM	Walking dog	15 minutes
	5:00 PM	Stretches, crunches	10 minutes

Exercise Boosts Endorphins

SOME FINDINGS REVEAL that individuals with chronic pain often have lower-than-normal levels of endorphins, which are powerful chemicals in the body that block pain signals and even provide pain-relieving power. Endorphins help to alleviate depression and anxiety, which are often associated with chronic pain. Exercising for 30 minutes a day is enough to increase endorphins in the body—and take advantage of the body's natural painkillers.

2. Stretching and Stabilizing Your Body

How often: Goal of 5 minutes, twice daily

The second category of Pain-Free exercises is daily stretching to keep your body flexible, balanced, and stabilized. These stretches will help to decrease pain and stiffness and will also help to keep your body balanced and prevent falls.

You might think that you're too strong to fall or if you do, your bones are strong enough to support the trauma without injury, but that's not always true. I have treated young adults who have suffered painful fractures after a fall. One young mother suffered a fall when she slipped down the stairs in her cotton socks. This fall resulted in two fractures that kept her from being active and caring for her three preschoolers. Another thirty-nine-year-old woman tripped on her son's bike and fell on her wrist. Again, a careless fall led to a painful fracture and weeks of rehabilitation. The incidence of falls increases with age and women are at higher risk if they have low bone density (osteoporosis).

Let's review the facts about falls:

- Falls are a leading cause of injury and fractures.
- More than 11 million older adults (1 out of 3) in the United States fall each year.
- One in 10 falls causes a serious injury.
- At least 95 percent of hip fractures nationwide are caused by falls. (The problem with hip fracture is that a quarter of those patients die within a year; 40 percent need a nursing home; and half who get to rehabilitation never walk without assistance again.)

As you learn the following stretching exercises, make a conscious effort to gently stretch your body. Overstretching or pushing too hard on a stretch can result in injury. You will need a long pole or broom handle for the first two exercises. After performing these exercises regularly for 3 weeks, you will notice a dramatic change in your flexibility and a reduction in pain.

Chest and midback: Place a long pole behind your back and across your shoulders, with your hands supporting the pole at each end. Then slowly rotate your torso to the left; repeat this movement in the opposite direction (see figure 2.7).

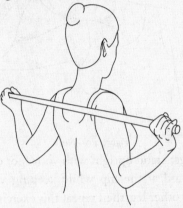

Figure 2.7—Chest and Midback

Shoulders: Hold a long pole with both hands over your head and slowly stretch from side to side, like a pendulum, several times. Then place the pole at shoulder level in front of you and gently turn to the right as far as its comfortable, then to the left. Repeat several times (see figure 2.8).

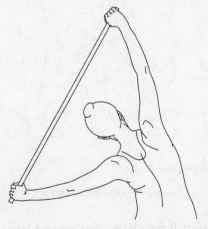

Figure 2.8—Shoulders

Neck: Place one hand on the side of your head just above your ear and gently push as if you are trying to touch your ear to your shoulder. Gradually build pressure while allowing no movement to occur. Hold and then relax (see figure 2.9).

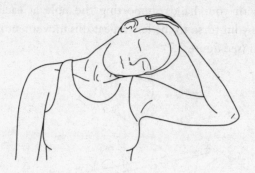

Figure 2.9—Neck

Legs and hamstrings: Stand upright with your foot on a bench or step. Slowly bend forward at the hip while keeping your back straight. Alternate with the other leg, then repeat this exercise. You will feel the stretch behind your thigh (see figure 2.10).

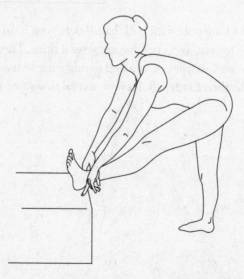

Figure 2.10—Legs and Hamstrings

Back: This exercise will help keep your posture straight and alleviate stress on your back and hips. Lie on your back with your knees bent, with your feet flat on the floor, hip-width apart. While contracting your abdominal muscles, press your lower back against the floor. You will feel your pelvis rock (tilt) toward your shoulders. The bottom of your buttocks and your pelvis will come slightly off the floor during the action (see figure 2.11).

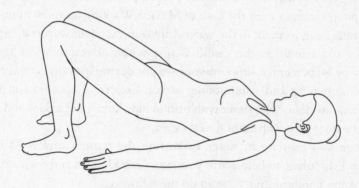

Figure 2.11—Back

3. Conditioning Your Body to Stay Fit

How often: Start gradually; work toward goal of 30 minutes of fitness exercises on most days of the week.

The third category of Pain-Free functional fitness exercises is conditioning. These exercises help your body stay strong, flexible, and fit with aging. While most people immediately think of jogging or high-impact aerobics as the optimal conditioning exercises, experts now believe that even moderate, daily exercise gives a tremendous benefit to overall function and health—as long as you are moving around and your heart rate gets a boost.

Walking Is Convenient

You can walk anywhere—at any time. You can walk in your backyard, in your neighborhood, at your workplace, at a local indoor mall, or even in place while watching a video. You don't have to buy a treadmill or drive to a fitness center to move your legs and walk daily. Findings show that walking just 5 minutes, 2 or 3 times a day, is a great start and will make a difference in the pain you feel if continued for a few weeks.

Obviously if you suffer with hip, knee, ankle, or foot pain, you will not stay with a walking program. Pain has a way of telling us when to quit exercising!

Biking or water exercises might be your exercise of choice, allowing you to burn calories, become fit, and also strengthen those key muscles that help support painful joints.

Water Exercise Supports Your Weight

Living on Florida's Gulf Coast, many of my patients have access to a swimming pool, a lake, or even the Gulf of Mexico. Working up to 30 minutes of swimming or movement in the water daily is an excellent way to strengthen muscles and condition the cardiovascular system. Because water reduces gravity by 80 percent, it supports your weight during movement and allows for strengthening and conditioning as you exercise. I recommend water exercises to patients who suffer with painful hips, knees, and ankles, and those with the deep muscle pain of fibromyalgia.

When you exercise in water, make sure the temperature is 83 to 88 degrees Fahrenheit, to help warm your muscles and joints and decrease pain. With water conditioning, you can do the following:

- Walk or jog in place, using a belt or life jacket to float without touching the bottom (I highly recommend this exercise as it's easy to do and convenient, and it works to get you in shape without increasing pain or adding stress on your joints).
- Stretch.
- Swim laps at your own pace.
- Use a kickboard as a flotation device.
- Hold on to the side of the pool (or a stationary object) and kick your legs.

PACE

CHECK WITH YOUR local YMCA for PACE classes (People with Arthritis Can Exercise) sponsored by the Arthritis Foundation. These water exercise classes are done in warm water, and focus on aerobic conditioning and full range of motion.

Gardening Counts as a Pain-Free Exercise

There are numerous household activities that qualify as exercise. For instance, many of my patients are avid gardeners and count this as their daily conditioning exercise. Gardening involves conditioning, strengthening, and range of motion—an all-in-one activity. Think about it! With gardening, you work all the muscles in the body as you walk, pull, lift, bend, stoop, dig, and even carry weighted objects (bags of potting soil, seed, and fertilizer, and so on). And, unlike other structured forms of exercise, it is difficult to stop gardening after 30 minutes—it's an activity that often continues for hours at a time and brings tremendous pleasure.

Of course, you don't have to be a gardener. The important thing is to choose exercises and activities that you enjoy—see a sample activities list on page 168. Then, make a firm commitment to do the exercise or activity most days of the week. I say "most days" because even the most energetic person needs to take a break every now and then. If you accomplish 5 or 6 days of exercise each week, I believe that you are doing quite well! If you exercise daily, the optimum goal, your weight loss and pain reduction benefit, may be even more noticeable.

START SLOWLY—BUT START NOW

If you are new to exercise after months of being sedentary, I suggest that you start slowly and pace yourself. Perhaps just begin with 5 minutes of one or two exercises a day. As you progress, add a few more minutes of exercise until you reach the goal of 30 minutes of exercise on most days of the week.

My patient Anna, age 58, had not exercised in months after fracturing her ankle when she slipped on her deck stairs. Even though the x-ray showed that the ankle was healed, Anna was afraid she would fall again. I convinced Anna that the more she moved around, the stronger her muscles would get and the steadier she would feel. Strong bones and muscles and a flexible body, are important to avoid falls—and fractures. I reminded Anna that as she began a walking regimen, she should feel no more pain or fatigue than when she started. She was to start slowly and gradually increase the exercise time to 30 minutes—not attempt to do 30 minutes the first day.

On day 1, Anna walked for 4 minutes around her backyard. The next two days, she repeated the same distance and felt more confident about walking. On day 4, Anna increased her walking to 7 minutes. She repeated the 7-minute walk on days 5, 6, and 7. On day 8, Anna again increased her exercise time to 10 minutes, walking around her neighborhood on the sidewalk. Within 4 weeks, Anna was walking 30 minutes every day. This feat changed

Anna's outlook on life, too. She was more confident, felt in control, and had no pain in her ankle. Also, Anna's mood was more upbeat and positive.

Again, you don't have to run for miles to make a difference in your pain threshold. Studies confirm that even a moderate exercise program reduces inflammatory responses in the body and helps fight the cellular damage of free radicals.

Start slowly—*but start now*. And continue to exercise moderately for long-term benefits.

Find Your "Energy" Time of Day

It's important to find the right time to exercise—a time when you feel alert and energetic, which helps make exercise easier and pleasurable. For example, many people like to jog in the evening after work. I usually run after I've seen my last patient. But most of my patients enjoy exercising in the early morning hours when they feel refreshed from a good night's sleep. Some of my patients jog with neighborhood friends before they go to work. Others go to a neighborhood Y to work out before showering and dressing for their workday. Many corporations have fitness centers on site, allowing employees to spend part of their lunch hour at the gym.

I'd like you to find that "energy" time of day that is right for you, and make a lifetime commitment to exercise every day at this time.

Select Activities You Enjoy

Review the following list of low-to-moderate-intensity exercises and activities, and select two or three that you enjoy. Alternate these activities throughout the week. Reaching your goal of 30 minutes of daily exercise will help you lose weight, decrease inflammatory markers that cause pain, and increase your overall cardiovascular and physical fitness.

Active play with children
Aerobics (low-impact)*
Badminton

Biking
Dancing
Dusting
Gardening
Golf (carrying clubs)
Hiking
Mall walking (3 mph)
Mopping floors
Stair climbing
Stationary cycling
Swimming (moderate)
Sweeping
Tae kwon do
Vacuuming
Walking (3 mph)
Washing windows
Washing your car
Water aerobics (moderate)

*Make sure your instructor is certified by the American Council on Exercise (ACE) or the Aerobics and Fitness Association of America (AFAA).

Pain-Free Exercise Goal

START SLOWLY AND build up to 30 minutes a day of conditioning exercise. You can do the 30 minutes all at once, or you can divide the exercise into two 15-minute segments or three 10-minute segments.

KAREN'S OSTEOARTHRITIS PAIN

Patient's name: Karen

Age: 55
Height: 5' 4"

Weight:	Before: 170	After: 150
Waist:	Before: 40	After: 35

Pain Quotient: Before: 9–10   After: 0–2

Favorite recipes: Cheesy Sausage Omelet, Pecan-Crusted Salmon, Egg and Olive Salad, Dr. McIlwain's Anytime Vegetable Soup

Favorite exercises: Walking, gardening, swimming laps, stretching

Symptoms: Karen had pain in her neck, knees, and hips for more than a year, with stiffness in the morning. She was fatigued and had difficulty getting started each day. In the afternoon hours, she could not concentrate at work and often depended on caffeinated drinks to stay alert. The caffeine then kept her awake at night so she could not relax and sleep.

Diagnosis: Osteoarthritis

After 16 weeks on the 4-step program: Karen lost 20 pounds and 5 inches in her waist. Her BMI decreased by more than 8 percent, and her high sensitivity C-reactive protein concentrations decreased by 35 percent. Karen was able to go off all medications while continuing to be very active with little pain.

MEREDITH'S FIBROMYALGIA AND DEEP MUSCLE PAIN

Name: Meredith

Age: 42
Height: 5' 2"

Weight:	Before: 140	After: 121
Waist:	Before: 33	After: 29

Pain Quotient:	Before: 10	After: 3

Favorite recipes: Hidden Yolk Scramble, Easy Edamame, Thai Cucumber Salad, Florida Orange and Spinach Salad

Favorite exercises: Stretching, yoga positions, swimming, range-of-motion exercises

Symptoms: Meredith told of having pain for five years in her neck, back, arms, and legs following an auto accident. The pain was constant and severe, with a pain rating of 8 out of 10. She said the pain awoke her at night, and she experienced fatigue and daytime sleepiness on most days. She had many medical evaluations and tried many medications without finding relief.

Diagnosis: Fibromyalgia syndrome

After 16 weeks on the 4-step program: Meredith lost 19 pounds and 4 inches in her waist. Her BMI decreased by more than 5 percent; her C-reactive protein concentrations decreased by 40 percent. Meredith rated her pain as 3 out of 10, and was able to exercise daily and enjoy her family and friends. She recently went back to work part-time as a preschool teacher.

ROSA'S RHEUMATOID ARTHRITIS AND INFLAMED JOINTS

Name: Rosa

Age: 36
Height: 5' 8"

Weight:	Before: 177	After: 152
Waist:	Before: 38	After: 32
Pain Quotient:	Before: 10	After: 2–3

Favorite recipes: Crispy Apples, Mixed Greens, and Gorgonzola; Multibean Salad, Apple–Butternut Squash Soup; Broccolini with Garlic and Ginger

Favorite exercises: Stretching, range-of-motion exercises, resistance machines at gym, swimming

Symptoms: Rosa told of having pain, stiffness, and swelling in her hands, wrists, elbows, shoulders, knees, ankles, and feet for more than two years. She was on many medicines but still awoke with stiffness that lasted 2 hours each morning. Rosa was tired all the time and she found it difficult to work and care for two children and her husband. Rosa was unable to exercise before starting the Pain-Free Diet. She also had difficulty taking medication because of gastrointestinal distress.

Diagnosis: Rheumatoid (inflammatory) arthritis

After 16 weeks on the 4-step program: Rosa lost 25 pounds and 5 inches in her waist. Her pain and stiffness improved greatly, and she was able to decrease her medications and exercise at the gym. Her C-reactive protein level dropped more than 50 percent.

MICHAEL'S LOWER BACK PAIN
AND DEPRESSION

Name: Michael

Age: 50
Height: 6'
Weight: Before: 249   After: 228
Waist: Before: 40   After: 36

Pain Quotient: Before: 8–10   After: 1–2

Favorite recipes: Apple and Oats, Spanish Omelet, Indian Rocks Broiled Seafood Kabobs, Buccaneers' Sloppy Joes, Thai Peanut Sauce (on french-style green beans)
Favorite exercises: Swimming, resistance exercises, yard work

Symptoms: Michael initially came to our clinic seeking treatment for low back pain due to a herniated disk. The pain limited his activity, and he was unable to exercise. He said he'd gained more than 40 pounds over the past five years and ate constantly because of the pain and from boredom. Michael had been on narcotic pain medication for several years and felt fatigued most of the time. He also suffered with depression and saw a psychiatrist.

Diagnosis: Back pain

After 16 weeks on the 4-step program: Michael lost 21 pounds in just 16 weeks. He lost 4 inches in his waist; his C-reactive protein level dropped 45 percent. He did his daily conditioning exercise in a heated swimming pool and was able to walk without pain after 3 weeks. He is now taking less medication and finds that his depressive symptoms have eased.

Keeping Bones Strong

WEIGHT-BEARING EXERCISE forces your body to resist gravity and stimulates cells in the body that make new bone. Strength training increases muscle strength, which increases bone strength. Strength training also increases flexibility.

SECRETS OF COMFORTABLE EXERCISE

Use Moist Heat Before and After Exercise

Almost all of my patients ask, "How do you exercise if you are in pain?"

I reassure them that there are easy ways to reduce the impact of movement on your muscles and joints so you can comfortably exercise without too much pain and stiffness. For instance, taking a warm shower, bath, or Jacuzzi soak, or using moist heat applications every morning and evening while you are on this program, can really make a difference. Heat is a superb soother of sore muscles and joints. It increases blood flow and helps to decrease inflammation and pain; moist heat, such as with a Jacuzzi or other whirlpool, is a highly effective way to apply this natural pain reliever. The warm shower or bath or moist heating pad eases aches, stiffness, and muscle spasms. As you use moist heat with exercise, your muscles will strengthen, making it easier to exercise more frequently and for longer periods of time.

When using moist heat, make sure it is not too warm, or you can burn your skin. It should feel soothing but not uncomfortable. If you have general body aches and pain, use the warm shower, bath, or Jacuzzi in the morning before exercise and again in the evening. If your pain is specific, such as shoulder, neck, hip, knee, or back pain, use a warm shower on the painful area or apply moist heat cloths or a heating pad for 15 minutes right before exercise, and then use the moist heat again on the same site immediately following exercise. Some of my patients initially find great relief when they do their exercises in a hot tub or sitting on a stool (with legs that have rubber tips, for safety) under a warm shower—one that is comfortable but not too hot. The constant heat flowing on the affected site helps to keep pain minimal and allows for easier movement.

Effective Types of Moist Heat

❑ Warm shower (sit on a shower chair, if needed)

❑ Warm whirlpool or Jacuzzi

❑ Hot packs (the kind that can be heated in a microwave)

❑ Warm, moist towel or cloth

❑ Moist heating pad

❑ Warm bath

❑ Heated swimming pool

❑ Disposable heat patch or belt (available at most pharmacies)

❑ Paraffin-mineral oil for hands and feet

❑ Terrycloth bag filled with flaxseed or rice (this can be heated in microwave)

Herbal Relief

If you need pain relief before and after a workout, try an herbal cream or salve. These can be found at health food stores and most drug stores:

Arnica (*Arnica montana*): The active components in arnica are *sesquiterpene lactones*, which are known to reduce inflammation and decrease pain. In ointment form, arnical tincture acts as an anti-inflammatory and *analgesic* for aches and bruises. Arnica may cause a skin rash in some people and should not be taken internally, as it can increase blood pressure and may damage the heart muscle.

Capsicum (*Capsicum frutesens*) (pronounced KAP-sih-kuhm): The ointment made from the spice in cayenne pepper is an effective treatment for muscle spasms, tension headaches, osteoarthritis and rheumatoid arthritis, fibromyalgia, or back or neck pain, and is also used to relieve pain caused by shingles and surgical scars. Capsaicin, the active ingredient in capsicum, temporarily stimulates the release of substance P in the nerves. This may initially result in pain and burning, but repeated applications deplete substance P, which limits the ability of the nerves to transmit sensations and reduces pain. It's best to use disposable gloves to apply three to four times daily, and if you feel you need to get it off, wipe the area with a dry cloth. If you wet the area, it may burn more. Wash your hands well after use to avoid getting in your eyes, nose, mouth, or private parts.

Capsicum is available as Capzacin and Zostrix, both are nonprescription drugs and are available at most pharmacies and grocery stores.

WHAT YOU CAN EXPECT

After engaging in a daily exercise program for 21 days, you will begin to notice a big difference in how you feel. Here are some of the immediate and long-term benefits you will enjoy:

- **Weight loss:** It will be easier to lose weight and also to maintain your goal weight with daily exercise.
- **Less pain:** Reduced weight means a reduction in pro-inflammatory markers, which reduces pain. When you weigh less, there is less pressure on painful muscles and joints.
- **More energy:** Aerobic conditioning boosts the amount of oxygen to your heart and muscles, which allows them to work longer. As your energy level increases, it will actually feel better to move around than to sit.
- **Activities are easier:** Daily living activities such as gardening, house-cleaning, or even carrying groceries from the car to your kitchen become easier when your body is fit. I have some patients who have fired their lawn services because they feel good again and enjoy being out-of-doors, working in their gardens.
- **Greater flexibility:** Flexible people have less risk of falling and being injured. You will carry your body with confidence and approach new situations without fear of tripping.
- **Stronger bones and muscles:** Physical impact and weight-bearing exercises help to keep bones strong and prevent osteoporosis (brittle bones) and painful fractures.
- **Improved sleep:** Exercise helps to increase the time you spend in deep "healing" sleep.
- **Healthier aging:** While research recently published in the *Journal of the American Geriatric Society* found that inactivity doubles the risk of mobility limitations as we age, daily activity has the opposite effect. In findings published in the journal *Neurology*, researchers concluded that exercise can slow cognitive declines, meaning boomers' minds can stay sharper longer.

Your Pain-Free Exercise Regimen

LET'S REVIEW THE various suggestions I've made for starting your Pain-Free exercise program. As you begin your program, checkmark the following items in this list. Then turn to pages 168 to 169 for suggested daily exercises given in the *Pain-Free Diet* menus for the first 28 days of the regimen.

_____ Review the list of activities and exercises on pages 168 to 169.

_____ Select two or three activities that you enjoy.

_____ Follow the steps on pages 151 to 159 to learn each of the functional fitness exercises. These exercises will help you to be more active throughout your day.

_____ With calendar in hand, pencil in a time each day to do these exercises and activities. I've given you a sample weekly calendar for Maura's back pain on page 160. Using this sample as a guide, add some exercises that will help your particular pain problem(s).

_____ Review the information about applying moist heat before and after exercise. If you need to purchase a moist heating pad, do so before you begin your exercise regimen.

_____ Talk to your physician about the exercise program before starting and ask if your medication is appropriate.

_____ Once you begin the exercise program, be sure to stop should you feel any unusual pain and call your doctor.

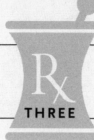

THREE

Stop the
Stress–Pain
Connection

Stop the Stress–Pain Connection

By learning to recognize the physical and emotional signs and symptoms of stress and deal with these in a positive manner, you can block the negative effects before stress triggers inflammation, pain, and illness.

IF YOUR PAIN has lasted for months, you may have forgotten what it was like to feel happy, carefree, and optimistic—even though you were a positive person before your pain began. Olivia's story is revealing of most people who live with pain:

"Two years ago I fell down a flight of stairs at work. After the fall, I remember feeling like electricity was shooting through my lower back, so much so that I was afraid to move my legs to stand up. I'd had mild back pain before, but this pain was frightening. Finally, some co-workers helped me to my feet, and I realized I could walk.

"A friend took me to a medical clinic nearby, and after doing an examination the doctor said that 'nothing was broken.' She told me to use moist heat on my back and take a nonsteroid anti-inflammatory drug to decrease inflammation and pain. The worst pain was over in about a week, but then it came back again—about one month later—and the moist heat and medications did nothing to alleviate it.

"The pain continued to haunt me every few months, and just anticipating the pain wore me down. My coping skills weakened, and I started to live in an emotional world filled with anxiety, fear, and some depression. When my marriage began to fall apart, I realized that the pain had crippled my ability to cope with life. The back pain literally controlled me, and I took my negative feelings out on my ex-husband, son, and co-workers."

Olivia suffered needlessly for months until she came to our clinic and started the Pain-Free Diet. A combination of weight loss, medication, and the relaxation strategies discussed in this step helped her regain control of her life—and her pain—and they can do the same for you.

There is no question that pain is emotional as it affects every part of your being. But now we are learning that emotions are linked to inflammation, just like your weight and your diet. In fact, in studies at Duke University Medical Center, researchers found that healthy people who have greater anger, hostility, and depressive symptoms have higher C-reactive protein levels than those individuals who are calmer. As I discussed on page 7, C-reactive protein is a marker of inflammation and strongly linked to obesity, pain, and serious illnesses.

This finding from Duke is not surprising, as many patients with pain also suffer with anxiety and depression. As an example, findings indicate that up to 42 percent of those individuals with rheumatoid arthritis have a depressive or anxiety disorder; from 14 to 23 percent of patients with osteoarthritis have significant levels of depression; and the frequency of major depression in those with fibromyalgia extends as high as 71 percent of patients. In my clinic, I find that patients with pain who are also depressed have significantly higher levels of pain, more painful joints, and overall poorer functional ability. These patients also tell of spending more days in bed than pain patients who are not depressed.

In this step, I want to delve into the serious problem of stress as the trigger of inflammation and pain. First, I will give you a simple quiz to let you analyze how frequently stress interferes with your life. Then I will explain the stress observation signs (SOS), or symptoms you might feel when your body is on high alert from too much stress. Once you can identify your stress observation signs, you can learn the suggested relaxation techniques that appeal to you and use these regularly to keep your body and mind in a calmer state. If you do use these relaxation strategies regularly, your body can be programmed to switch into a meditative, calming state before the impending stress affects you physiologically. The goal you want to achieve is a consistently much calmer mind and body, which will help to reduce inflammation and pain.

Understanding the Pain-Stress Connection

I realize that the stress of living with pain or even worrying about your pain returning can put you into emotional overload. Pain can affect your mood and cause irritability, impatience, and higher levels of frustration. However, while pain is a physical problem, emotional fears and other stress factors play an overall role in the experience. For example, there may have been a time when you cut your finger, but did not feel pain until you looked at the finger and saw blood. At that moment, the finger probably began throbbing as you became aware of the injury. Similarly, just the anticipation of pain causes an increase in heart rate and quickens breathing (both symptoms of stress). But learning how to relax offers a real potential to reduce the physical strain and emotional, negative thoughts—and increases your ability to self-manage stress.

What Is Stress?

Simply stated, stress describes the many demands and pressures that all people experience each day. These demands may be physical, mental, emotional or even chemical in nature. The word *stress* encompasses for us both the stressful situation known as the stressor, and the symptoms you experience.

Feeling *stressed out* is a term we all use to describe the impact of life stressors. When you're stressed out, you feel increased anxiety, moodiness, distractibility, and a host of other physical symptoms listed on page 187. But as a pain sufferer, your stress is different and greater than someone who does not have pain. Not only is the pain itself a physical stressor, but you may encounter social stressors with loss of friends and activities, work stressors with difficulty working or even loss of job, and family stressors with feelings of resentment or dependency on others. You may also have to deal with waiting for doctors' appointments, financial distress because of medical bills or loss of income, and feelings of anger, irritability, frustration, and loneliness because you have no control over any of this.

HOW DOES STRESS AFFECT MY PAIN?

Stress results in high levels of cortisol in the body, which can increase heart rate, blood pressure, LDL cholesterol and triglyceride levels. Without cortisol, you could not possibly survive an emergency, as it literally gives you super-energy in the form of blood glucose and causes other changes in the body that help the "fight or flight" stress response. In other words, it keeps you pumped so you perform optimally at the time.

But when cortisol levels are elevated for a while, that creates a gradual and steady cascade of harmful physiological changes to the body, including suppression of the immune system, which is associated with the development of many diseases. For instance, extensive studies show that the death of a spouse is often associated with an elevated mortality rate for the survivor, particularly in the early periods after the loss. There is also a relationship between psychological stress and the increased risk of colds. When study volunteers were given nasal drops containing one of five cold viruses, colds and cold symptoms increased, depending on the amount of psychological stress.

Stress also influences the onset of inflammatory diseases such as arthritis and specific types of pain (back, neck, muscle). Given all the scientific evidence, it makes sense to presume that decreasing stress can alter body chemicals to help modulate pain. Yet for many people, the negative stress cycle can be difficult to interrupt. These individuals live daily with back or neck pain, which is often a result of their stress response. Some of my patients suffer with chronic tension headaches—or even migraines—when life's stressors overwhelm them. I also have patients with inflammatory arthritis, such as rheumatoid or lupus, who have much more joint pain, swelling, and stiffness when they are experiencing overwhelming stress than when their lives are calmer.

Too Much Stress Increases Waistlines

When cortisol levels remain high, this causes abdominal fat to accumulate—evidenced by an increased waistline and the "apple" body shape. We're now learning that people who have apple body shapes have an increased risk of diabetes, cardiovascular disease, and pro-inflammatory markers. Some findings indicate that the relationship between waistline size (called central fat) and inflammation may be more significant than the connection between total obesity and inflammation.

Regardless of your weight or waistline size, chronic or long-term stress itself also produces pro-inflammatory cytokines. So when stress continues for days to weeks, it weakens the immune system and increases inflammation. In fact, studies show that individuals who feel tremendous job stress, particularly those who harbor feelings of burnout, have high inflammatory responses in the body.

Mitch, age 48, had been slim most of his life until his brokerage firm took a financial hit a few years ago. In less than a year, Mitch's business lost thousands of dollars and he had to lay off twenty-four employees. During this period, Mitch gained 19 pounds and 4 inches in his waist—because he could not stop eating. "Every time the stock market would fall, I'd drink another milkshake or two and snack nonstop when I got home at night. I wasn't hungry but I literally could not stop eating. I guess the food must have filled an emotional void."

Mitch said he started a liquid diet to lose the weight quickly, and that resulted in more feelings of overwhelming stress. "Even though I was sticking with the weight-loss plan, I felt ill at ease and anxious, and had a hard time sleeping. I had to go off the diet so I could get along with my wife and kids, and function normally at work."

Yes, dieting, too, can add stress to a person's life. It's even possible that this diet plan may increase your stress, at first. There aren't many people who can adapt to a new style of eating—not to mention a reduction in calories—without feeling a bit anxious. We know that when the body is deprived of calories or "favorite foods," our brain's reward system kicks in, causing us to crave some foods (probably other foods not on this diet, too!). For example, my female patients usually tell of craving sugar/fat combinations (chocolate chip cookies and rich desserts), whereas my male patients say they crave protein/fat combinations (hot dogs, double cheeseburgers, and pepperoni pizza). This brain reaction involves changes in dopamine and endorphins, two chemicals that are also involved in drug addiction, which explains why the cravings can be so strong and difficult to resist.

That's why it's even more important to realize your personal signs of stress and learn the relaxation therapies to reduce these signs before the chronic stress results in illness or pain. To help you reduce stress as you follow the Pain-Free Diet, I encourage you to go slowly—don't try to lose all the weight in a few weeks or months. Make this a lifetime proposition—not a "quick fix." I recommend that patients plot their weight loss in intervals—such as, "I'd like to lose 10 pounds by (date)_____." Or, "I'd like to lose 5 or 10 percent of my weight by (date)_____." I find that when my patients can lose 10 to 15 percent of their initial weight and maintain this loss for a year or longer, that this is an exceptional medical result—even if the patients do not ever reach their "ideal" weight as dictated by height/weight charts or BMI calculations. Setting short-term weight loss goals, you can easily meet will also help reduce any additional stress of following a diet.

Chronic Stress Can Lead to Depression

Alicia had lived for years with chronic back pain that resulted from an automobile accident in her early twenties. Now thirty-five, this mother of twin girls said she felt malaise most of the time. "Even when my back pain is minimal, I still feel highly anxious and have a low mood," she told me. "It's been so long since I felt upbeat that I have honestly forgotten what it feels like to enjoy life."

I started Alicia on a newer antidepressant, a selective serotonin reuptake inhibitor (SSRI), and within days, she noticed an improvement in her mood. She's been on the medication for more than a year now, and reports that family and friends continually comment on her upbeat personality. Not only does she feel more relaxed and hopeful, but the medication helps her to sleep well at night and feel more alert during the daytime hours.

Serotonin is a neurotransmitter in the body linked to mood. When serotonin levels are increased in the brain, it is associated with a calming, anxiety-reducing effect, and in some cases, with drowsiness. But studies show that too much stress or pain can lead to permanently low levels of serotonin, which can result in ongoing anxiety and depression. Researchers believe that abnormal levels of serotonin and other neurotransmitters, chemical messengers in the brain, are some of the primary causes of mood disorders such as depression.

Depression is associated with many chronic illnesses. When they are in pain, patients become ever more focused on their inability to exercise and be active, and on their personal suffering. The many appointments with physicians to try to find relief, combined with the cost of these attempts, and episodes of painful flare-ups, add to this frustration.

As time goes on, those who suffer with unmanaged pain can have trouble keeping a job; the absences become too frequent. If income is reduced or lost altogether, this adds to the financial stress for the patients and their families. The stress of dealing with loss of income, along with the pain, can cause relationship problems with loved ones and friends.

Over time, the longer pain goes unmanaged, the more likely the person will experience feelings and notice signs caused by the stress, which can make the pain worsen and create even more problems, including:

- Difficulty sleeping, leading to constant fatigue
- Inability to exercise, resulting in poor aerobic and physical fitness

- Difficulty concentrating from the side effects of medications, leading to poor performance
- Increased irritability, from lack of sleep or medications' side effects
- Withdrawal from favorite activities, because of low energy
- Changes in appetite, due to medications
- Depression

There is a better way to live. Using the suggestions in this step, you can end a depressive cycle and rediscover an active and exciting life.

How Stressed Out Are You?

THINK BACK OVER the past few weeks. Check the stress symptoms you have experienced:

_____ I feel tired or run down.

_____ I get angry or frustrated easily.

_____ I have lost interest in my work.

_____ Stress bothers me more now than before.

_____ I get headaches or stomachaches regularly.

_____ I have trouble sleeping.

_____ I feel depressed or unhappy frequently.

_____ I have lost my sense of humor.

_____ I have become more rigid and critical.

_____ I feel overwhelmed or overworked.

_____ I frequently use mood-altering drugs or alcohol.

_____ I clench my jaws while sleeping.

_____ I have lost or gained weight recently.

If you experienced more than two or three of these symptoms, you need to work on your stress-coping skills. Continue to read this step for insight and ideas to hep you recognize your stress signs and relax—to reduce your pain.

IDENTIFYING YOUR STRESS OBSERVATION SIGNS (SOS)

Emotional stress can trigger a host of health-related problems, ranging from memory loss to impaired immunity; it definitely plays a role in pain. However, thanks to extensive research, scientists have a better understanding of how stress affects the body. The fact is *stress is simply a pain trigger.* Whether there will be health consequences after a stressful episode depends on *your responses* to the external event. These responses involve the immune system, the heart and blood vessels, and how certain glands secrete hormones that help regulate various functions in the body, such as brain function and nerve impulses. All of these responses interact and are profoundly influenced by one's coping style and psychological state.

Review the *Stress Observation Signs* (SOS) on page 189, and determine the particular ways your body responds to life's stressors. These reactions are well-documented symptoms that occur with the "fight-or-flight" response; the initial stress response that happens automatically when you feel threatened. When the mind perceives a threat, the pituitary gland at the base of the brain responds by stepping up its release of adrenocorticotropic hormone (ACTH). The burst of ACTH is followed by a flood of stress hormones such as cortisol, epinephrine (adrenaline), and norepinephrine (noradrenaline) that pour into the body to help you respond in a hyperalert, quick manner.

When the stress has passed, epinephrine and norepinephrine subside and return to normal levels. But cortisol continues to stay elevated, especially in those over age forty. And elevated cortisol over a period of time results in excess abdominal fat and pro-inflammatory markers.

In short, stress does not cause pain but, rather, your response to stress can increase your reaction to pain. By learning to recognize the physical and emotional signs and symptoms of stress and deal with these in a positive manner, you can block the negative effect before they cause you to have increased inflammation and pain or become ill.

25 Common Stress Observation Signs (SOS)

CHECK THE FOLLOWING symptoms that you experience with chronic stress:

1. Anger
2. Anxiety
3. Apathy
4. Asthma
5. Back pain
6. Chest pains or tightness
7. Depression
8. Headaches (including migraines and tension headaches)
9. Heart palpitations
10. Hives
11. IBS (irritable bowel syndrome)
12. Insomnia
13. Inability to relax at night
14. Inability to concentrate
15. Irregular menstrual periods
16. Jaw pain
17. Loss of sexual desire or function
18. Mood swings
19. Neck pain
20. No energy
21. Rapid pulse
22. Rashes
23. Short temper
24. Short-term memory loss
25. Weight loss or gain

Stress and Chronic Illness

A LARGE PROPORTION of all visits to doctors' offices are for stress-related complaints. Along with pain, stress is linked to an increased risk of the following diseases:

- Allergies, asthma, and hay fever
- Back and neck pain

- Cancer
- Heart disease
- High blood pressure
- Migraine headaches
- Peptic ulcer disease
- Stroke
- TMJ (temporomandibular joint) syndrome
- Tension headaches

Accepting Your Pain

Your ultimate goal is to get the point where you can accept your pain, and then start making modifications to handle it in your life. The opposite of acceptance is denial, and this behavior will work against any pain rehabilitation efforts. It is vital to accept that issues such as anger, anxiety, and loss of self-esteem can affect your pain. An interesting study of patients with pain found that higher levels of acceptance were associated with less attention to the pain, greater commitment to daily activities and social affairs, higher motivation to complete activities, and greater confidence rating personal performance of daily activities.

LEARNING TO RELAX
AT THE FIRST SIGN OF PAIN

When my patient Susan feels her neck pain coming on, she drops whatever she's doing at the time, turns on her favorite CD, and begins her deep abdominal breathing exercises (page 194) that put her in a calmer state of mind. If Susan is at home, her teenagers know to leave her alone for a while until she has finished her relaxation exercises and calmed her body and mind. If she's at work, Susan closes the door to her office and takes her phone off the hook to allow a break from the frenetic workplace environment.

Learning to drop what you're doing and relax at will in the midst of having pain is not an easy skill. Nevertheless, Susan and many of my patients have found ways to interrupt the pain process whenever they feel the first sign of tension or pain in their muscles and joints.

While many of my patients use relaxation therapies to remove themselves mentally and emotionally from the painful moment, pain is extremely complex. Not only is it influenced by changes in your body chemistry, there are environmental, psychological, and social triggers. Chronic pain is not like an ear infection, where you can take an antibiotic and, in a few days, there's no more pain. There is no salve or ointment that can cure it. Many times, your doctor cannot even find what's causing the pain. Unlike a fracture or a known disease, soft-tissue pain may not appear on an x-ray or even respond to medical treatment. Moreover, how do you measure pain? What may be horrible pain to you may be considered mild to your colleague, or vice versa.

Calm the Mind to Calm the Body

Because pain is so elusive and difficult to measure, it lends itself well to mind/body therapies. I have found in my clinic that relaxation therapies are extremely effective in decreasing pain when used in conjunction with moist heat applications (page 174) and medications. Often when patients take pain medications over a long period of time, their bodies adjust to that level of medication. However, when my patients combine stress management and relaxation therapies along with pain medications, most report having fewer episodes of debilitating pain and some patients even take less pain medication. When they add moist heat applications (or hot baths or showers) to the medications and relaxation therapies, they experience even greater results with less pain and increased mobility. Although no one is sure just how relaxation exercises work to decrease pain, some researchers believe that muscle relaxation might reduce the number of pain signals delivered to the nervous system.

Change Your Pain Perception

There are some studies showing that we can learn how to make our brains feel less pain and react to pain so that it doesn't bother us as much or even at all. Surely you've heard stories of a person who can walk on nails or hot coals without feeling pain. I recall reading about a mother who virtually lifted a car off her teenage son when the jack collapsed on him while he was changing a tire. Another recently reported story was of the young surfer in Hawaii who felt no pain when her arm was taken off by a shark. Likewise, the soldier in Iraq who miraculously never stopped in his effort to save his buddies even with a severe injury to his leg, claimed to feel no pain.

While these efforts used to be thought of as heroic, scientists can now show some of the brain responses with the use of magnetic resonance imaging (MRI) of the brain using special techniques. This functional neuroimaging allows pain volunteers to see their brain activity while feeling pain. As they try to control the pain using various mind/body methods, the volunteers can then see how this changes brain activity.

Just thinking about your pain—creates pain. This is why relaxation therapies can help you regain control.

Start with Simple Strategies

Moving beyond acceptance of your pain, it's time to learn some easy ways to relax and regain control of your life. For example, evaluating your priorities and budgeting your time are excellent organizational skills that can help you eliminate the "clutter" in your daily life. Saying no when you are overly committed is another positive strategy you can take—even though most people have a difficult time doing this. I remember one patient, Marianne, telling me that simply getting the nerve to say no to family and friends caused her more inner turmoil than actually saying no!

Exercise Boosts Mood and Restful Sleep

A super way to de-stress includes increasing exercise. Regular exercise increases the neurotransmitter serotonin, helping to boost mood and regulate sleep. Exercise also increases phenylethylamine, a natural stimulant that also boosts a positive sense of well-being. In addition, as I discussed in Rx #2, exercise keeps your joints moving in a full range of motion and keeps your muscles and bones strong—all important for living pain free.

Reduce Caffeine

I also encourage my patients who have difficulty coping with stress to greatly reduce their caffeine intake, as this food mimics the stress response with a short-term rise in their blood pressure and heart rate. Many patients have come to my office and found their usually normal blood pressure and pulse elevated after having a cup or two of coffee. Caffeine also heightens the side effects of pain medications, resulting in feelings of trembling or high anxiety for some individuals.

RELAXATION TECHNIQUES

Along with lifestyle strategies to reduce stress, there are several relaxation therapies that are scientifically substantiated to speed production of new immune cells and control the damaging stress hormone cortisol.

For example, deep abdominal breathing helps *reduce* physical stress and negative thoughts—and *increases* your inner ability to self-manage pain. Visualization allows you to remove yourself mentally from a stressful moment and lower your anxiety, heart rate and blood pressure. With biofeedback, you work with a trained therapist to understand your SOS before they cause injury to the body. Music therapy can be done anyplace, anytime, as you relax and reduce muscle tension.

Each of the following relaxation strategies helps to ward off and even control painful flare-ups that can be triggered by stress. If practiced regularly, your body will learn to elicit the relaxation response, which can help to relieve the added anxiety that often accompanies ongoing pain. Many people find that it is only after several weeks of daily, consistent practice that they can maintain the relaxed feeling beyond the practice session itself, so don't give up before you see the benefits.

Try to set aside a period of 10 to 15 minutes that you can devote to relaxation practice, removing any outside distractions that can disrupt your concentration. You might even start with only 2 to 3 minutes and gradually increase as your skills improve. Recline comfortably so that your whole body is supported, and relieve any muscle tension. Use a pillow or cushion under your head, if this helps.

Caffeine in Foods

Coffee, drip	5 oz.	90–115 mg
Coffee, perked	5 oz.	60–125 mg
Coffee, instant	5 oz.	60–80 mg
Coffee, decaf	5 oz.	2–5 mg
Coffee, espresso	1.5–2 oz	100 mg
Coca-Cola	20 oz	60 mg
Coke, Diet	20 oz	80 mg
Tea, 5 min. steep	5 oz.	40–100 mg

Tea, 3 min. steep	5 oz.	20–50 mg
Herbal tea	8 oz	0 mg
Hot cocoa	5 oz.	2–10 mg

Deep Abdominal Breathing

Remember Susan, my patient who uses deep abdominal breathing to gain control over her neck pain? Breathing is one of the few activities of the body that we can consciously control. The problem is that increased stress tends to result in improper breathing—from the upper chest, using the muscles of your neck and upper back. This shallow breathing results in an increase in your blood pressure and heart rate. On the other hand, breathing slowly from your abdomen allows more oxygen to fill the lungs and brain, resulting in less anxiety, reduced upper-body tension, and even lower blood pressure.

Deep abdominal breathing actually alters your psychological state, making a painful moment diminish in intensity. Think about how your respiration quickens when you are fearful or in great pain. Then take a deep, slow breath and feel the immediate calming effect, reducing both stress and levels of pain.

Researchers know that the brain makes its own morphinelike pain relievers, called endorphins and enkephalins. These hormones are associated with a happy, positive feeling and can help relay "stop pain" messages throughout your body. During deep abdominal breathing, you will oxygenate your blood, which triggers the release of endorphins, while also decreasing the release of stress hormones and slowing down your heart rate.

Lie on your back in a quiet room with no distractions. Place your hands on your abdomen, and take in a slow, deliberate deep breath through your nostrils. If your hands are rising and your abdomen is expanding, then you are breathing correctly. If your hands do not rise, yet you see your chest rising, you are breathing incorrectly. Inhale to a count of 5, pause for 3 seconds, and then exhale to a count of 5. Start with 10 repetitions of this exercise, and then increase to 25, twice daily. Use this exercise any time you feel anxious or stressed because of pain.

Blowing Your Stress Away

HERE'S A STRESS-REDUCTION technique that I share with my patients: Buy a bottle of inexpensive children's bubbles (in the toy section at any store), and use it to learn how to breathe slowly. Breathing from your abdomen, blow through the bubble blower with a steady stream of breath. If you blow too hard or too softly, you won't get any bubbles. However, you will find that smooth and steady breaths will produce a nice flow of bubbles. Use this breathing technique without the bubbles when you are feeling stressed.

Progressive Muscle Relaxation

Carla suffered with the deep muscle pain of fibromyalgia for three years until she learned progressive muscle relaxation. This young mother had tried several pain medications, but these made her tired and unable to care for her two preschoolers. Desperate for relief, Carla agreed to learn the relaxation therapies in this step and found progressive muscle relaxation especially helpful when her muscle pain flared up in the evening hours, keeping her from relaxing or sleeping.

This exercise involves contracting and then relaxing all the different muscle groups in the body, beginning with your head and neck and progressing down to your arms, chest, back, stomach, pelvis, legs, and feet. To do this exercise, you focus on each set of muscles, tense these muscles to the count of 10, then release to the count of 10. Go slowly as you progress throughout your body, taking as long as you can. Get in touch with each part and feel the tension you are experiencing. Notice how it feels to be tension-free as you release the muscle.

Studies show that when you can create a strong mental image using this type of relaxation technique, you actually feel "removed" from cumbersome stress and the pain response. This mindfulness, or focusing all attention on what you feel at the moment, can help you move beyond the pain you may feel as you become centered in a world of health and inner healing.

Visualization

Most people look forward to vacations because it gives the body and mind respite from the frenzied pace of everyday life. But who can afford to take time off from work to drive to the mountains or seashore every time life's stressors engulf them? For most of us, we'd have to leave town every Friday night in search of serenity! But that's the beauty of visualization. This form of relaxation is used for controlling emotional distress and pain. While some people are naturally better at imagining than others, I believe that most people can learn this simple technique and then use it anytime their SOS (page 188) become apparent.

Simply thinking about your pain can create more pain, which is why relaxation therapies such as visualization can help reduce pain. To practice visualization, take a time-out in a quiet environment without distractions. During this time, try to visualize a peaceful, relaxing scene, perhaps a vacation spot you have enjoyed—a photograph of a mountain sunset, soft, pink clouds in a light blue sky, or an early morning sunrise at the beach. Focus on this scene in your mind, and try to recapture the moment as you imagine the sounds, smells, textures, and feelings you would experience. As you visualize the serenity of the scene, become mindful of your breathing and anxiety level. If you still feel tense, breathe deeply from your abdomen to increase relaxation. Don't let outside stimuli interrupt your imagery time.

Once you have learned how to relax with visualization, keep a picture or photograph of the scene with you. If you sense that your SOS are increasing, take time apart from whatever you are doing and visualize the peaceful scene. Again, try to re-create the calmness of the scenic moment as you create your own circle of serenity.

Optimism Eases Pain

JUST AS SCIENTISTS have found that positive beliefs can ease pain (the placebo effect), they also have found that negative beliefs and influences can induce pain (the nocebo effect).

Music Therapy

Many successful businesses have found that background music—particularly classical music, such as works by Mozart—is especially effective in helping clients relax. I find that music is an excellent means of reducing mental stress as well as physical pain. In clinical studies, both doctors and patients agreed that listening to music produced greater decreases in peaks of tension and greater compliance with relaxation practice.

Try to spend 10 to 15 minutes a day listening to soothing music. Once you've achieved this habit, add another mind/body technique, such as visualization or deep abdominal breathing while listening to music. Does the music help you feel more relaxed? I find it helpful if the pace of the music is slower than your heart rate, or approximately 60 beats a minute, as this can encourage your heart rate to slow down. Some studies have shown that music can also lower blood pressure, while also reducing levels of stress hormones.

Massage

Along with mind/body therapies to de-stress, massage helps to relieve depression and anxiety, an increase in the number of natural "killer cells" in the immune system, lower levels of the stress hormone cortisol, and reduced difficulty in getting to sleep. For those who have neck or back pain, massage therapy can help relax sore muscles and increase mobility. This form of drug-less therapy has also been shown to increase circulation, give relief from musculoskeletal pain and tension, act as a mind/body form of stress release, increase flexibility, and increase mobility.

Biofeedback

There is good evidence that biofeedback might help to relieve many types of pain, including tension and migraine headaches, according to a consensus statement from the National Institutes of Health. This therapy is based on the idea that when people are given information about their body's internal processes, they can use this information to learn to control those processes. In one study by researchers at the University of South Alabama, 80 percent of children who suffered with migraines were symptom-free after receiving intensive biofeedback training. In other research, some headache patients who were able to increase hand temperature using thermal biofeedback, also experienced fewer and less intense migraine headaches.

With biofeedback, you are connected to a machine that informs you and your therapist when you are physically relaxing your body. Using sensors placed over specific muscle sites, the therapist will read the tension in your muscles, heart rate, breathing pattern, and the amount of sweat produced or body temperature. Any one or all these readings can let the trained biofeedback therapist know if you are learning to relax.

Over time, the ultimate goal of biofeedback is to learn to relax outside the therapist's office when you are facing real stressors. If learned successfully, electronic biofeedback can help you learn how to control your heart rate, blood pressure, breathing patterns, and muscle tension when you face pain or stress—even when you are *not* hooked up to the machine.

Meditation

Meditation involves sitting still in a quiet place while placing your ultimate focus on the moment. During this time of personal solitude, you let all the day's worries leave your attention and only experience the moment. Meditation is believed to result in a completely "free" mind while affording you a chance to recover from the day's pain, interruptions, and stress. Because pain is a complex interaction between sensations, thoughts, and emotions, meditation can help self-regulate the pain you feel and increase your ability to handle stress.

Meditative techniques are a key element in the Arthritis Self-Help Course at Stanford University. More than 100,000 people with arthritis have taken this course and learned meditation-style relaxation exercises. Graduates report a 15 to 20 percent reduction in pain.

To learn to meditate, find a quiet place indoors or outdoors with no distractions. While sitting in a comfortable position, close your eyes and focus on your breathing, keeping it very slow and intentional. You should notice the sensation of air passing in and out of your nostrils during this moment of solitude. It's difficult to reach the stage of complete "mindfulness," where your thoughts are focused entirely on the moment instead of your past or future. But as you practice this repeatedly, you will learn how to focus on your breath, which will keep your mind from wandering. After 10 to 15 minutes, stop the meditation and return to your normal activity.

Yoga

I have many patients who are interested in yoga for exercise purposes and also for managing their daily stress. This ancient discipline originated in India more than four thousand years ago, and is quite popular in the United States. Hatha yoga, the most commonly practiced branch used in the West, emphasizes specific postures, active and relaxation poses, breath control, concentration, and meditation.

If practiced regularly, yoga can relieve muscular tension or pain by improving range of motion, relaxing tense muscles, and increasing muscle strength. Practicing yoga when you are feeling anxious may help to reduce stress when you are on the job or at home. In fact, findings show that, for some, just three months of weekly yoga training results in an increase in physical well-being, significant improvements in perceived stress, and a marked reduction of headache and back pain. Yoga also reduces blood levels of cortisol, which is important for reducing inflammation, as discussed on page 4.

There have been several recent studies on yoga and pain, and the findings are all encouraging:

- In one study, researchers concluded that yoga was effective at improving function and reducing back pain and the benefits persisted for at least several months.
- Another study revealed that yoga improved carpal tunnel syndrome after just three weeks of practice.
- A revealing study of patients with rheumatoid arthritis found that hand grip strength of both hands increased in patients following yoga practice.
- Perhaps the most intriguing findings are on the effect of yoga on body weight, blood pressure, and insulin resistance. In one study, just 8 weeks of yoga practice resulted in 1.5 to 13.6 percent reduction in body weight, while even relatively short-term practice of yoga was found to reduce blood pressure. More than ten studies that evaluated the effects of yoga on markers of insulin resistance show significant improvements.

Of course, there are dozens of other studies, but the point is that alternative therapies like yoga can be extremely healing for pain sufferers.

Practicing a simple pose known as corpse pose is an easy and relaxing way to meditate. The more you practice meditation in this pose, the easier it will become to quiet your mind. With time, the practice of meditation becomes more calming and you will feel more rejuvenated.

1. Lie on your back on a comfortable surface, and stretch your arms and legs out straight. Keep your arms down by your sides, and extend your legs straight from the hips. Your feet should be about 12 inches apart, with both feet turned out slightly to keep the feet, ankles, and legs relaxed.

2. With palms facing upward, keep your arms 8 to 10 inches from the body. Lengthen your back on the floor and feel all your muscles stretching and releasing.

3. Notice your shoulder blades and hips, and adjust the body until you feel balanced on both the left and right sides of your body. Scan your body and consciously relax every muscle group, including your throat, face, and eye muscles. Continue this scanning as you lie down and relax, and become aware of areas in which you might hold chronic tension.

4. As you lie there, feel the breath take you into a deeper relaxed state.

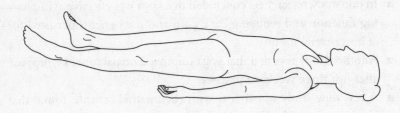

Figure 3.1—The Corpse Pose

Increase Your Social Network

Having intimate relationships with family and friends helps us to feel accepted and maintain optimism and aids in stress management. All of these emotional benefits lead to stronger immunity, which is vital to staying well and functioning optimally. In fact, it is well documented that people who are happily married and/or have large networks of friends not only have a greater life expectancy compared with those people who do not, but they also have fewer incidences of just about all types of disease.

Support groups such as those sponsored by the Arthritis Foundation are geared toward meeting the unique needs of those who suffer with pain. Although support groups are not psychotherapy groups, they do provide patients with a safe and accepting environment to vent their frustrations, share their personal stories, and receive comfort and encouragement from one another. In many such groups, the latest medications are discussed and coping suggestions are shared among members. Assurance is given that someone else knows what you are going through as people share their struggles in living with pain. After joining a support group, you may realize that the best experts on treating pain are those men and women who live with it daily, although it still remains critically important to talk your doctor before trying any treatment suggested by other patients in the group.

I have listed support organizations for individuals with different types of pain on pages 262 to 265. You can call or write to these organizations for literature, or check out their Internet sites. These groups are focused on educating consumers about pain-related disorders, along with giving the latest methods to diagnose, treat, and prevent pain.

On a different note, social support does not have to be just with other people. You might form emotional attachments with your animals. I have many patients who live alone yet find comfort and camaraderie with a pet—an attachment that is every bit as strong as that between a parent and a child. There are countless papers published in the area of animal-human bonding revealing the health benefits of this type of interaction.

Interestingly, even having a plant can be beneficial. In a study at Yale University, researchers found that when people had a plant present in their room they had speedier recoveries compared with people who did not. I have patients who live alone yet are positive and optimistic about their lives because of a connection to their gardens. These patients find meaning and purpose from being outdoors and enjoy the healing benefits of nature.

CALMING HERBAL THERAPIES

If you try the relaxation therapies yet still need help calming down, talk to your doctor about medications that may help to boost your mood or ease your anxiety. If you are opposed to taking medications to ease stress, then ask your doctor about the following herbal therapies.

St. John's Wort

St. John's wort (*Hypericum perforatum*) is used by millions to ease mild to moderate depression. In Germany, more than 20 million individuals use St. John's wort.

Recently, German researchers have found that St. John's wort was as effective as such SSRIs as Prozac (fluoxetine) but without any serious side effects. In one study published in the journal *International Clinical Psychopharmacology*, volunteers who took either St. John's wort or the antidepressant fluoxetine were evaluated by psychiatrists for symptoms of depression. After 6 weeks of treatment, researchers concluded that those individuals who took St. John's wort reported fewer and less serious side effects. For instance, just a few participants in the St. John's wort group reported mild gastrointestinal complaints. Yet those volunteers who took fluoxetine reported far more serious symptoms, such as dizziness, tiredness, anxiety, and erectile dysfunction. The researchers concluded that St. John's wort clearly is superior as the medication of choice for mild to moderate depression in both effectiveness and safety, when compared to fluoxetine.

St. John's wort is available as capsules, tincture, extract, oil, and dried leaves and flowers. St. John's wort can cause sensitive skin in sunlight. (Caution: Since the mechanism of action of St. John's wort is uncertain, do not use it with antidepressants such as monoamine oxidase inhibitors and SSRIs. Pregnant women are also not advised to take St. John's wort.)

Chamomile

Chamomile (*Matricaria recutita*) depresses the central nervous system and may also aid in boosting immune power. This healing herb is said to increase relaxation, promote quality sleep, and can be used to relieve nervousness, upset stomach, and menstrual cramps.

Chamomile is available as dried herb, supplements, and herbal tea. This herb may cause problems for those allergic to ragweed, although there are no reports of toxicity.

Passion Flower

Passion flower (*Passiflora incarnata*) provides a mild tranquilizer effect and helps to ease insomnia, stress, and anxiety.

This herb is available as tincture, fruit, dried or fresh leaves, or capsules. Avoid combining passionflower with prescription sedatives, and do not take if pregnant or nursing.

Valerian

Valerian (*Valeriana officinalis*) has a sedative effect and has been shown to help in treating insomnia. It is also used to relieve high anxiety, stress, and nervousness.

Valerian is available in capsules, tincture, and dried flowers. Avoid taking valerian if you already take prescription antidepressants; it may cause stomach upset.

Selecting Quality Supplements

Plants can vary greatly in their potency, and there is no government regulation for ingredients in herbal remedies. How do you know which supplements are effective? When choosing herbs, look for the ones labeled "standardized." This means the manufacturer measured the amount of key ingredients in the herbal batch, so the chances are greater that you will get what you pay for in a "standardized brand." Also, buy herbs from a reputable manufacturer instead of an off-brand that may be cheaper. Some of the known brands include General Nutrition, Natrol, Sundown, and Nature's Bounty, among others. You might ask your pharmacist to recommend a reputable brand.

If you decide to take herbal supplements, be sure to talk to your doctor, pharmacist, or a certified nutritionist about side effects. Herbal therapies are not recommended for pregnant women, children, the elderly, or those with compromised immune systems. In addition, some herbs have sedative or blood-thinning qualities, which may dangerously interact with NSAIDs or other pain medications. Others may cause gastrointestinal upset if taken in large doses. For example, ginkgo biloba may cause nausea, diarrhea, stomach upset, and vomiting if taken in larger doses, and may reduce clotting time. Anyone taking coumadin should not take this herb. If you are taking drugs with a narrow therapeutic index such as cyclosporine, digoxin, hypoglycemic agents, lithium, phenytoin, procainamide, theophylline, tricyclic antidepressants, and warfarin, you should avoid herbal products altogether. In addition, St. John's wort, which is taken by many for the treatment of depression, may cause serious herb–drug reactions, particularly if taken with SSRI agents.

WHAT YOU CAN EXPECT

Experiment with the different mind/body therapies until you find those that help you to relax at will. It might take several weeks of practice, but you can find relaxation strategies that can help calm the stress response by slowing your heart rate and breathing, modulating your mood, and helping you to feel relaxed and stress-free. Use the therapies of choice throughout your day, particularly at known stressful times such as driving in traffic (use deep abdominal breathing). Also use the therapies that work best for you during the evening, especially before going to bed, to increase relaxation and induce restful sleep.

As coping with any chronic condition can have psychological consequences, I highly recommend to my patients that they seek professional counseling periodically, especially if they are having problems coping with stress or the pain itself. For instance, cognitive behavioral therapy is a popular approach that helps you to challenge negative thought patterns and feelings of helplessness. Talk therapy can help you to learn appropriate and workable coping strategies to deal with everyday stressors, your personal relationships, and any problems of daily living. Studies show that psychotherapy can actually change parts of the brain, resulting in a long-term improvement in the mood problem.

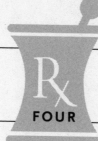

FOUR

Increase the Quality of Your Sleep

Increase the Quality of Your Sleep

Learning these helpful, practical sleep strategies will help ease your pain, calm nighttime anxiety, and let you get healing, quality sleep.

Y OU LIE IN bed for what seems like hours, tossing and turning, trying to find a comfortable position so that your hip or shoulder or back does not ache. Finally, the pain medication your doctor prescribed begins to work; you relax and slowly fall asleep. As you enter the dream stage, you unconsciously roll over on your side—the wrong side. Like an electric shock, the pain penetrates throughout your entire body, sending a red-alert signal to your brain, letting you know that it has not yet retreated .

Now you lie in bed—again wide awake—while you pamper your pain by propping up on pillows, trying to find a comfortable position that will allow you to rest. You count sheep, take your pulse, go over your to-do list for the next day and become even more aware of the minutes ticking by on your bedside clock. After an hour, you doze off and sleep restlessly the rest of the night until dawn when your alarm rings. You realize you must awaken—this time to start your day feeling very irritable and unrefreshed . . . and still in pain.

If there's one coexisting problem almost every pain sufferer shares, it is an inability to sleep well at night and feel refreshed and alert the next day. Whether from difficulty finding a comfortable position, waking up throughout the night because of neverending pain, or experiencing nonrestorative, light sleep, most pain sufferers agree that they are "tired of feeling tired" and want pain-free solutions to guarantee refreshing sleep.

Lucy's Fibromyalgia

Lucy's sleep problem was so serious that she told me that she dreaded going to bed each night. This forty-seven-year-old administrator suffered with the deep muscle pain of fibromyalgia, along with symptoms of anxiety, mild depression, and difficulty sleeping.

"I lie awake much of the night and then feel fatigued the next day," Lucy said at her first consultation. "Lately, I wake up feeling as if I hadn't slept at all, even though I was in bed for eight to ten hours. At work, I have an increasing inability to concentrate, making it impossible to be effective and focus on my deadlines."

Lucy finally came to our clinic because she was so exhausted that she had dozed off while driving home from a visit with her elderly mother. Luckily, the car hit some speed bumps on the side of the road, which startled her awake, and she was able to drive home safely. It was at that time when she called our clinic. Lucy knew she needed medical help.

PAINFUL SLEEP: MORE THAN A NUISANCE

Almost all patients with pain suffer from sleep problems and the resulting daytime sleepiness and fatigue. Ron, a forty-one-year-old former professional soccer player, said he had not slept more than 2 or 3 hours a night for weeks. While that sounds exaggerated, I'm sure he was basing that on the way he felt each day: fatigued, weary, and irritable with an inability to concentrate or be productive at work. Ron wanted relief—now. But before he could begin to sleep well, I explained that he had to deal with his pain problem. As you probably know, if you are in pain at night, it is virtually impossible to relax and sleep well.

In this last step in your Pain-Free program, I want to help you solve the problem of pain interfering with your sleep. I'll explain how inflammation and obesity are both linked to quite serious sleep disorders such as obstructive sleep apnea (OSA), a problem in which the person literally stops breathing many times throughout the night. OSA is increasingly common among many overweight patients who also suffer with pain.

Because lack of sleep is now thought to decrease the level of serotonin in the body (a brain neurotransmitter that contributes to a relaxed mental state and also plays a role in the pain that you feel), I will unravel these findings so you can see how the sleep-pain-inflammation puzzle fits together—especially in your situation. Finally, I want you to sleep—tonight! So I'll suggest some helpful, practical sleep strategies that have worked for my patients and will help you relax your mind and body, ease your pain, and finally get healing sleep.

A century ago, Americans used to sleep an average of 10 hours each night. But that was before Thomas Edison perfected the incandescent lightbulb in 1880. Since then, the number of hours Americans sleep has greatly declined. When you add the addictive power of television, home video, and high-speed Internet, is it any wonder that the average American today only sleeps 6½ hours? According to the National Sleep Foundation, the proportion of adults in the United States sleeping less than seven hours per night has increased from 16 to 37 percent over the past forty years. Not only can lack of sleep put undue stress on the body, it can result in physiological changes that increase your pain, affect your cognitive skills and job performance, increase inflammation in the body, and even seriously disrupt your breathing at night.

The Stages of Sleep

STAGE 1: Light sleep

STAGE 2: Moderate sleep

STAGE 3 AND 4: Deep sleep, called delta sleep

STAGE 5: REM (rapid eye movement) sleep, the dream stage

Increases in Pain and Moodiness

Many different pain ailments are associated with sleep disturbances. But researchers are not certain if the sleep problem causes the increase in pain or if the pain itself causes the sleep disorder.

There are five stages of sleep (see sidebar, above). REM (rapid eye movement) sleep, during which we dream, is associated with psychological well-being and feeling refreshed upon awakening. People who are deprived of REM sleep complain of irritability and moodiness. Stages 3 and 4 appear to be the most important for physical recovery. If sleep disturbances occur during these stages, you will wake up feeling tired and may complain of muscular aches and pains.

About twenty years ago, scientists in Toronto, Canada, discovered that patients with fibromyalgia syndrome had stages of sleep that were contaminated by an "alpha rhythm," the normal brainwave of a person who is *awake*—not asleep. In the study, researchers showed that healthy volunteers deprived of delta sleep (the deepest stage of sleep) by being exposed to noise, also developed periods of deep sleep mixed with alpha waves, again like those brainwaves seen in wakeful states. Interestingly, when deprived of delta sleep, these people experienced musculoskeletal discomfort and mood symptoms similar to those of the patients with fibromyalgia. These findings suggest that this sleep interruption itself may have contributed to the achiness or pain and mood symptoms. Your body needs deep sleep to repair itself.

Poor-quality sleep also leads to lower levels of serotonin in the body. Serotonin is a naturally occurring neurotransmitter (brain chemical) that is associated with a calming, anxiety-reducing feeling in the body. When serotonin is depleted from lack of sleep, the result is an *increase in sensitivity to pain*, as well as increased feelings of anxiety, malaise, and even depression. There are also studies showing that a decrease in serotonin triggers an increase in appetite, particularly for carbohydrates such as candy, pastries, and other baked goods.

Decreases in Alertness and Performance

Not only is sleep deprivation associated with increased pain or decreased pain tolerance, it causes changes in other mental functioning. If you are sleepy during the day, this can lower your concentration and lessen your short-term memory. Your energy, productivity, and attention to detail are all compromised. Some patients who suffer with night after night of sleep loss because of pain often ask if they have attention deficit disorder (ADD), a problem that is associated with an inability to focus or pay attention, and sometimes with impulsive behaviors.

For instance, perhaps this is coincidence, but I find it unsurprising that both the Chernobyl and Three Mile Island nuclear disasters occurred in the early morning hours, when the body wants and needs sleep. And while most people think that a captain's drunkenness caused the Exxon *Valdez* oil spill, the National Commission on Sleep Disorders says otherwise. The real problem may have been the severe fatigue of the ship's third mate, who was in charge at the time of the accident.

Activities that involve total concentration, such as driving a car, are much riskier because of the tendency for a sleep-deprived person's attention to wander without diversion or constant stimulation. I find it interesting that the National Commission on Sleep Disorders concluded that drunk driving causes fewer fatalities than does sleepiness. In fact, the National Sleep Foundation estimates that 100,000 traffic accidents and 1,500 fatalities occur each year due to driver fatigue. Studies reveal that the day following the switch to daylight savings time, when an hour of sleep is lost, traffic accidents *increase* by 7 percent. When we later gain the hour back going off daylight savings, we see the opposite—a 7 percent *decrease* in traffic accidents.

Increases in Appetite and Weight

A recent study of healthy volunteers in the medical journal *Sleep* found that those who slept 2 to 4 hours a night were over 200 percent more likely to be obese than those volunteers who got 7 hours of sleep. In fact, one study found, just a 16-minute loss of sleep per night also increased the risk of obesity.

These studies indicate that sleep loss lowers the level of leptin, a hormone that stimulates metabolism and decreases hunger. Sleep loss or shorter hours of sleep appear to boost the concentration of the hormone ghrelin, which increases hunger.

In a study of middle-aged women, researchers concluded that weight gain was related to the amount of sleep each night. This study started about twenty years ago when more than 68,000 women were asked every two years about their sleep patterns as well as their weight. After sixteen years, the findings revealed that those women who slept 5 hours or less each night weighed 5.4 pounds more than the women who slept 7 hours. The researchers thought that the women who slept less were not only threatened by weight gain but by obesity, as well. For instance, women who slept 5 or less hours per night were 15 percent more likely to become obese than were women who slept 7 hours each night.

In line with these studies, there is increasing evidence that people who sleep less than 6 or 7 hours a night have a higher risk for diabetes. Researchers at the University of Chicago found that losing just 3 to 4 hours of sleep over a period of several days is enough to trigger metabolic changes that are consistent with a prediabetic state. The body's ability to keep blood glucose at an even level declines significantly. This may be because sleep deficit affects the immune function of the body. In one study, scientists found that a 45 percent reduction in total sleep time resulted in a nearly 30 percent reduction in cellular immunity. Getting quality sleep is now considered a basic defense mechanism to staying healthy and preventing disease.

Reductions in Levels of Human Growth Hormone

We now know that as deep sleep decreases, so does the secretion of human growth hormone. By the time a person is thirty-five, this can decrease by as much as 75 percent. Studies have shown that this hormone deficiency can lead to obesity, loss of muscle mass, and a reduced capacity to exercise.

We want to do everything in our power to promote deep sleep and the production of growth hormone, so overweight baby boomers with chronic pain can lose weight, reduce inflammation and pain, and be active again.

Inflammation and Obstructive Sleep Apnea (OSA)

When you lose sleep (even just an hour a night), pro-inflammatory chemicals are markedly increased in the body, resulting in pain. Now some experts believe that there is a possible link between OSA and inflammation.

Snoring is caused by the vibration of the soft parts of the throat while breathing in and out during sleep. OSA involves periods of breath-holding while snoring. The periods of stopped breathing are called apneas, which are caused by obstruction of the upper airway. Apneas may be interrupted by a brief arousal that does not awaken you completely—you often do not even realize that your sleep was disturbed. Yet if your sleep was measured in a sleep disorders laboratory, technicians would record changes in the brain waves that are characteristic of the arousals.

Obstructive sleep apnea results in low oxygen levels in the blood, because the blockages prevent air from getting to the lungs. The low oxygen levels also affect brain and heart function. OSA is more common than asthma in adults, and up to two-thirds of the people who have obstructive sleep apnea are overweight.

For those who have OSA, elevated levels of pro-inflammatory markers in the body can directly worsen of the problem. Those with more than twenty apneas (complete obstructions) per hour of sleep may have a greater risk of dying from cardiac rhythm and rate disturbances, and complications of high blood pressure such as stroke and heart attacks, than do people with fewer apneas.

Common Symptoms of Obstructive Sleep Apnea

- Morning headaches
- High blood pressure
- Dry mouth
- Sore throat upon awakening
- Depression
- Concentration problems
- Memory failure
- Impotence
- Excessive daytime sleepiness
- Restless sleep (increased movements)
- Choking sensations
- Frequent awakenings
- Irregular heart rhythm

PAIN-FREE SLEEP STRATEGIES

I realize that you didn't open this book to only learn about the problems associated with being overweight. You need answers—and you need them today! Millions of pain sufferers have disordered sleep, especially insomnia (difficulty falling asleep or maintaining sleep, or an inability to feel rested despite adequate time spent in bed). With age, the prevalence of insomnia increases as sleep time decreases, even though the time spent in bed might increase. There is a better way.

Here are some easy strategies that I recommend to my patients when they are "tired of feeling tired" and want to make changes to increase quality sleep.

Lose Weight

I've said it repeatedly throughout this book—weight loss is the best way to guarantee pain-free living. Not only does carrying around extra baggage increase pressure on your joints, weighing as little as 10 or 15 pounds over your desired weight can increase pro-inflammatory markers which worsen problems like obstructive sleep apnea. Following the Pain-Free Diet will help you lose pounds and reduce the risk.

Find a Comfortable Sleep Position

Trying to find a comfortable sleep position with pain is not easy—but it can be done. Here are some suggestions:

Make sure your mattress is firm for good support during sleep. If you are sleeping on a soft mattress, this puts extra stress on your back, neck, and hips. In addition, if your mattress is more than three years old, consider replacing it with a new, firm mattress. Some of my patients who suffer with arthritis, disk disease, fibromyalgia, and other problems with pain prefer sleeping on a waterbed, and find that it gives maximum support and comfort.

Try a pillow. If your neck, shoulders or upper back causes you pain problems, try one of the specially made pillows that fit the contour of your neck and ease stress on that part of the body. You can find these online or at any medical supply store.

If you have back pain, including arthritis of the spine, try to sleep on your stomach for at least a brief period each night. This can help to prevent posture problems, particularly a "stooped over" appearance, which is a common problem in many types of spinal arthritis, especially ankylosing spondylitis (see glossary).

Take a Warm Bath before Bedtime

Sleep characteristically occurs when the body temperature is declining, whereas wakefulness occurs when the temperature is rising. In findings published in the journal *Clinical and Sports Medicine*, researchers concluded that skin temperature of hands and feet (particularly warm feet) seems to be the crucial variable for the association between internal body temperatures, sleepiness, and sleep. You can safely take advantage of skin warming/core cooling by taking a luxurious warm bath before bedtime to enhance sleepiness and deeper sleep and keeping your bedroom temperature cool (about 68 degrees Fahrenheit).

Keep Your Bedroom Dark and Quiet

Wear earplugs if you are bothered by noises while sleeping. Some people find that "white noise"—from a machine that produces a humming sound or a radio tuned to a station that has gone off the air—helps. Also, get black-out shades for your room to make sure it is fully dark. Light is a cue for the body to awaken; darkness signals relaxation and sleep. Wear a sleep mask if you are ultrasensitive to light and find it disrupts your sleep time. Turn your clock with the face toward the wall so you are not tempted to check the time all night long.

Watch What You Eat and Drink

Eating foods high in complex carbohydrates can raise levels of serotonin, a brain chemical essential for sound sleep. Also, try eating foods rich in B vitamins, such as whole grains, peanuts, bananas, and sunflower seeds, which help to counteract the effects of stress. Lastly, avoid alcohol and caffeine. Alcohol can cause you to fall asleep quickly, but many people wake up in the middle of the night and have trouble getting back to sleep. Even one cup of coffee (150 mg of caffeine) can disturb the quality of sleep, increasing wakefulness and making it difficult to feel rested the next day.

Consider Taking Melatonin

The natural hormone melatonin may be helpful for many who have difficulty falling asleep. Melatonin is thought to regulate sleep cycles and help to set the brain's biological clock. But the amount of melatonin produced by the body *lessens as we age*, with adults experiencing about a 37 percent decline in daily melatonin output between the ages of twenty and seventy. We know that melatonin is a potent free radical scavenger, and melatonin deficiency is related to suppressed immunocompetence.

Melatonin supplements are sold over-the-counter at most pharmacies; talk to your doctor and see if this might help your sleep problem. Some people who take melatonin find it helps them fall asleep easily; others wake up after several hours of deep sleep and are unable to get back to sleep.

Maximize Sleep with Yoga

The Child's Pose, shown below, can be done several times a day. This is a great yoga posture to practice as you prepare for sleep, or if you need a calming moment in a stressful day.

Kneel on the floor on your hands and knees with your hands under the shoulders and your knees under your hips, with your toes touching. Stretch your neck forward and lengthen your spine through the tailbone. Gently rock the weight of your body back toward your feet, letting your hips stretch further back as you continue to lengthen and stretch your spine. Stretch your arms forward and walk your fingertips as far forward as they will go on the floor or rug, lengthening your arms fully. Stretch from your shoulders.

As your hips stretch backward, focus on the stretch from your armpits to your hips, lengthening the sides of your torso and back. If you are flexible, continue stretching and relax your neck as your forehead touches the floor. Pressing the forehead against the floor or pillows helps to calm your mind as the forehead and eye muscles completely relax. If this is hard, put one or two pillows under your forehead. Rest a few seconds and allow your forehead and eye muscles to relax.

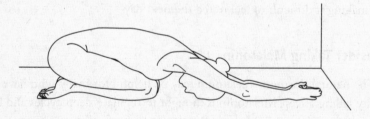

Figure 4.1—The Child's Pose

Avoid Naps

If you are exhausted, a short nap might help you to become more alert. But for most people, napping only makes it more difficult to get quality sleep at night. If you do nap, keep it to around 20 minutes so you will sleepy again at bedtime.

Avoid Nighttime Exercise

It is known that people who exercise close to bedtime have more problems relaxing and sleeping. This may be because exercise is stimulating, causing you to feel alert and raising your body temperature. The raised temperature will only begin to fall as long as 5 or 6 hours after exercise, and this fall signals to the body that it is time to sleep. Try to exercise early in the day while you have energy or in the afternoon, so your body has time to calm down before you climb in bed.

WHAT YOU CAN EXPECT

Using the various strategies in this step, you can find the right combination that eases your pain, relaxes your mind and body, and allows you to sleep 7 to 8 hours a night. Your goal should be to sleep undisturbed and pain-free throughout the night and awaken feeling rested and ready to take on the day.

Sleep is often interrupted by pain and is hard to improve, even with sleep medications. The lack of sleep can be frustrating, and this alone can increase feelings of fatigue, anxiety, and even more pain. After a night of poor sleep, you may suffer with increased stiffness in the muscles and joints, which can take hours to alleviate.

Using the Pain-Free Sleep strategies in this chapter, I believe that you can make a difference in the quality—and quantity—of your sleep. If you are still having sleep problems, talk to your doctor about one of the new nonaddictive sleep medications for short-term use.

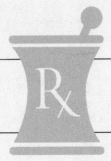

More Ways
to Fight Pain

How to Relieve
Common Pain Problems

MORE THAN 70 million Americans suffer with pain every day. Using the four steps in the Pain-Free Diet along with medications recommended by your physician, you can alleviate the pain associated with the following specific problems, and be sure your muscles and joints work well many years from now.

- Back pain
- Osteoarthritis
- Fibromyalgia
- Neck pain
- Rheumatoid arthritis
- Gout
- Systemic lupus erythematosus
- Bursitis and tendinitis
- Disk disease
- Knee pain
- Hip pain
- Foot pain
- Sports injuries
- Carpal tunnel disorder

Back Pain

More than half of all Americans suffer with back pain each year. Usually, the back pain is acute and lasts from 3 to 7 days at a time. But when back pain doesn't go away for weeks to months at a time, it can become constant, severe, and limiting. Back pain is one of the most common causes of disability, especially in men and women under age forty-five, and the number-one occupational hazard.

The most common source of back pain is from the muscles, tendons, and ligaments around the lower spine, but pain can affect any part of the back or neck. It is extremely common to have osteoarthritis (wear-and-tear arthritis) in the spine that shows up on x-rays. Back pain can also occur after injuries, with fibromyalgia syndrome (page 224), and even after a fracture in one of the bones of the spine (most commonly from osteoporosis). If your back pain lasts more than a few weeks, it is important that you check with your doctor to be sure no other medical problems are causing the pain.

The pain in the lower back may travel down one or both legs (sciatica), especially if there is pressure on the sciatic nerve in the lower spine. The chronic pain often results in nighttime awakening, making good sleep impossible. The constant pain is usually hard to control even with medications and is a constant source of stress, limiting activities and the ability to work. The lower activity level can lead to weaker muscles, an irritable mood, and depression. Those who suffer from back pain know how limiting it can be and how it affects every part of one's life.

If you have back pain plus any of the following warning signs, call your doctor immediately:

- Pain that travels down one or both legs
- Pain that is worse with a cough or sneeze
- Pain that awakens you at night
- Changes in your bowel or bladder habits
- Fever or weight loss
- Pain in your abdomen

Treatment Plan for Back Pain
- Apply moist heat twice daily to affected area (or bathe in a warm tub of water or use a Jacuzzi)

- Do neck, hip, and back exercises (pages 153 to 159)
- Focus on stretching and strengthening muscles
- Do crunches to strengthen abdominal muscles
- Swim to strengthen muscles, increase endurance and end fatigue (start slowly and increase gradually over time)
- Work on quality of sleep and stress control
- Lose weight (see Rx #1 of the Pain-Free Diet plan)
- Talk to your doctor if medications are needed

Osteoarthritis

Osteoarthritis or the "wear-and-tear" arthritis, is the most common type of arthritis, affecting about one-third of the adults in the United States. Osteoarthritis usually happens after overuse or injury to a joint, especially in joints that support weight over the years (the knees, hips, and back). Although osteoarthritis can occur in younger adults in their twenties, it is more common in those over age fifty. Overweight individuals and those with injuries to joints or a family history of osteoarthritis have a higher risk of getting this painful ailment.

With osteoarthritis, the cartilage that cushions a joint gradually wears away, resulting in pain with movement of a joint. You may feel some stiffness in the morning that wears off in a few minutes. If you have pain or stiffness that lasts more than a few weeks in your knees, back, hands, neck, or other joints, check with your doctor for an accurate diagnosis.

Treatment Plan for Osteoarthritis:
- Apply moist heat twice daily on affected areas
- Do back, neck, hip, and shoulder exercises (pages 153 to 159)
- Do stretches daily to keep body balanced and flexible
- Walk or swim daily to improve endurance and end fatigue (start slowly and increase gradually over time)
- Ride a stationary bicycle if you have osteoarthritis of the knees, hips, or ankle (to avoid added pressure on these joints)
- Work on quality of sleep and stress control
- Lose weight (see Rx #1) and stay on the Pain-Free Diet to reduce inflammation
- Talk to your doctor about medications to ease pain and inflammation

Fibromyalgia

Fibromyalgia is an arthritislike ailment that causes intense pain everywhere—the back, neck, arms, and legs. In fact, if there are not many areas of pain involved, then it is not typical fibromyalgia.

The severity of the pain may vary from day to day. However, in most cases, the pain is relentless, with fatigue that can be as severe and limiting as the pain itself. With fibromyalgia there is also morning stiffness, poor sleep (often, the pain awakens the sufferer), anxiety and depression, difficulty concentrating, headaches, irritable bowel syndrome with abdominal pain, diarrhea or constipation, urinary burning and frequency, restless legs, mouth dryness, and swelling and tingling in the hands, along with the typical trigger points over the body. For most patients with fibromyalgia, the pain and fatigue interfere with their career, their family responsibilities, and all their personal relationships. The patients' frustration is made worse by the fact that they do not look sick or injured, so most family and friends simply do not understand why there is so much limitation and pain.

Fibromyalgia is much more common in women than men. Although the exact causes of fibromyalgia are not known, it sometimes follows an injury or illness and may be related to the body's malfunction in pain processing. This malfunction causes the patient to be more sensitive to pain and the pain lasts far longer than normal.

There are no tests to accurately diagnose fibromyalgia. A doctor will make the diagnosis after a physical examination, patient discussion, and laboratory tests to rule out other more serious diseases.

Treatment Plan for Fibromyalgia
- Apply moist heat twice daily on affected areas
- Do neck and back exercises (pages 154 to 155)
- Do stretches beginning on page 163 to keep your muscles flexible
- Walk daily to improve endurance and end fatigue (start n slowly and increase gradually over time)
- Work on quality of sleep and stress control
- Lose weight (see Rx #1) and stay on the Pain-Free Diet to reduce inflammation
- Talk to your doctor about medications to ease pain and help with anxiety and sleep problems

Neck Pain

The most common cause of neck pain comes from pain and inflammation in the muscles and other soft tissues around the neck. This can happen gradually or suddenly and is most common along with osteoarthritis in the neck. The pain can be severe and limiting. The important thing is to check with your doctor to be sure there are no other serious causes of the neck pain. Osteoarthritis, rheumatoid arthritis, disk disease, or other medical illness might be present and may need early treatment to be successful.

If your neck pain hurts when you cough, or travels down one or both arms; if you notice weakness in the muscles of your arms; or if the pain awakens you at night, then you should make an appointment with your doctor as soon as possible for further evaluation.

Treatment Plan for Neck Pain
- Apply moist heat twice daily to affected areas
- Do neck, back, and shoulder exercises (pages 153 to 159)
- Stretch daily, using the exercises beginning on page 163
- Lose weight (see Rx #1) and stay on the Pain-Free Diet to reduce inflammation
- Reduce stress in the neck and shoulders if you feel muscle tension
- Work on sleep quality
- Talk to your doctor about medications to ease pain, if needed

Rheumatoid Arthritis

Rheumatoid arthritis affects more than 10 million Americans and is more common in women than men. Although this painful illness is more common between the ages of twenty and fifty, young children and older adults can develop rheumatoid arthritis.

The symptoms of rheumatoid arthritis can come on gradually or suddenly. Oftentimes there is stiffness on arising in the morning that may last several hours. Fatigue can be extremely limiting, sometimes more limiting than the pain itself. Although rheumatoid arthritis can cause permanent damage and deformity in up to 70 percent of cases, it is very treatable.

Rheumatoid arthritis occurs when the immune system goes haywire and in an inflammatory reaction, attacks the linings of the joints. This type of arthritis causes pain, swelling, and stiffness in the joints of the hands, wrists, elbows, shoulders, knees, ankles, and feet. The exact trigger, whether a virus, an inherited gene or other cause, is not known. But once the inflammatory reaction starts, the lymphocytes (one variety of the body's white blood cells) cause the release of cytokines, messengers that trigger more inflammation and destruction. These reactions happen in the joints but can spill over to other areas of the body.

The most important cytokine in rheumatoid arthritis is tumor necrosis factor (TNF), but others are being discovered that can also cause damage. TNF triggers many destructive enzymes. New medications have been developed to block TNF; some have been shown to control the pain and swelling, improve fatigue, and actually stop the joint destruction in rheumatoid arthritis.

After a physical examination, discussion other laboratory tests and x-rays, your doctor can make an accurate diagnosis. Specific markers in blood tests, such as *rheumatoid factor*, C-reactive protein, sedimentation rate, and other protein studies help shape this diagnosis.

Treatment goals include controlling the pain and stiffness and preventing long-term damage to joints. Although these goals can be achieved with current treatments, it is best to start treatment early to prevent joint damage.

Treatment Plan for Rheumatoid Arthritis
- Apply moist heat twice daily to affected areas
- Do hand, wrist, elbow, shoulder, knee, ankle, and foot exercises (pages 153 to 159); also, talk to your doctor or a physical therapist for recommended exercises
- Stay on the Pain-Free Diet)
- Avoid foods that might trigger inflammation (see page 110)
- Find sleep strategies that will increase quality and quantity of sleep
- Take prescribed medications and see your doctor regularly for follow-up visits to assess your arthritis

Gout

Gout is a type of arthritis caused by excess uric acid in the blood, resulting in an accumulation around the joints. Over time, the body produces excess uric acid, excretes less than usual, or both causing the level of blood uric acid to gradually increase. At times these joint deposits can trigger attacks of severe inflammation with pain, swelling, warmth, and redness around the joint.

Gout most commonly involves one joint, usually the first toe. The attacks are sudden and painful with touch or movement, such as experiencing severe pain with even the weight of bedsheets. Blood tests and an examination of a small sample of joint fluid can confirm the diagnosis of gout. NSAID medications, colchicine, or a cortisone medication can help the acute gout attack resolve in just a few days.

Treatment Plan for Gout

- Lose weight (see Rx #1) and stay on the Pain-Free Diet to reduce inflammation
- Avoid animal products and alcohol
- Take NSAIDs (see page 235)
- Talk to your doctor about colchicine or another medication to quickly resolve the gout attack
- Take prescribed medications such as allopurinol to help prevent further attacks

Lupus (Systemic lupus erythematosus, or SLE)

This inflammatory type of arthritis causes joint pain, swelling, stiffness, and fatigue, and is most common in women ages twenty to forty. In about 20 percent of patients, rashes are common, including a facial rash over the cheeks called a "butterfly rash." Many patients are sensitive to sunlight, which can worsen the rash. Hair loss and sensitivity to cold exposure in the hands and feet (a condition called Raynaud's phenomenon) can occur. Most important is the possibility of internal organ disease, most common in the kidney but possibly affecting any organ.

Blood tests can help confirm *Systemic lupus erythematosus (SLE)*. About 95 percent of all cases have a positive *antinuclear antibody (ANA)* test, although many with a positive blood test do not actually have SLE. Once the diagnosis is made then proper treatment can start, but it is very dependent on which problems of SLE are present. Most cases are controlled without long-term damage to internal organs, but patients need regular medical follow-up to monitor internal organ function.

Treatment Plan for Lupus

- Apply moist heat twice daily to affected areas if arthritis is a part of the pain problem

- Lose weight (see Rx #1) and stay on the Pain-Free Diet to reduce inflammation
- Use relaxation techniques (Rx #3) to control stress response
- Find sleep strategies that help to increase quality and quantity of sleep
- Take prescribed medications and see your doctor regularly

Bursitis and Tendinitis

With bursitis, the sac through which a tendon or muscle moves becomes inflamed, causing extreme pain with movement or pressure. Bursitis is common in the shoulder and the hip but it can happen in many other areas of the body.

Tendinitis occurs when a tendon attaching a muscle to a bone becomes inflamed, often from repetitive or excess use. Common types of tendinitis include "tennis elbow" or "golfer's elbow," resulting from overuse in these activities. The shoulder and heel are also common areas to be affected. Tendinitis can happen along with another type of arthritis, such as rheumatoid arthritis, osteoarthritis, or fibromyalgia.

Treatment Plan for Bursitis and Tendinitis
- Apply moist heat twice daily to affected areas
- Avoid additional repetitive stresses to injured area
- Lose weight (see Rx #1) and stay on the Pain-Free Diet to reduce inflammation
- Take prescribed medications (talk to your physician)

Disk Disease

In disk disease, the cartilage disk that is the cushion between two vertebral bones becomes weak, and the contents of the disk protrude to cause pressure on a nerve coming from the spine. This happens most commonly in the lumbar spine of the lower back, resulting in lower back pain and pain that travels down one or both legs. It can also affect the middle, upper back, or neck portions of the spine. The cause of the disk disease is thought to be degeneration of the disk material, but it can be triggered by injury.

Your doctor will make a diagnosis by using an x-ray and a magnetic resonance imaging (MRI) or computerized tomography (CT) scan. The pain is treated with pain medications, rest, and heat, along with gradually resuming exercise. Surgery is needed in about 10 percent of cases.

See your doctor if the pain is worse with coughing or sneezing. If the pain awakens you at night or if you have weakness in a leg or numbness or a tingling sensation down your leg, call your doctor. Also, if you experience difficulty controlling your bowel movements or your bladder, let your doctor know this immediately. In these cases, there may be pressure on nerves that must be treated quickly for best results.

Treatment Plan for Disk Disease
- Apply moist heat twice daily to affected area
- Do range-of-motion exercises (see pages 153 to 156) for the back, neck, and knees twice daily
- Lose weight (see Step 1) and stay on the Pain-Free Diet to reduce inflammation
- Monitor your stress and sleep habits
- Take prescribed medications (talk to your physician)

Knee Pain

Pain in one or both knees that lasts more than a few weeks or is severe needs medical evaluation. The most common causes of knee pain are osteoarthritis or bursitis, which can be very painful and limiting. If your knee locks in one position or it buckles or gives way when you step, there may be a problem with the cartilage or ligament in the knee. Check with your doctor for proper diagnosis of the problem so that treatment can begin.

For knee pain due to osteoarthritis, the Pain-Free Diet and exercises are the most important and effective treatments. If other problems are present, your doctor can make an accurate diagnosis and prescribe proper treatment or medication.

Treatment Plan for Knee Pain
- Apply moist heat twice daily to affected area
- Do exercises (pages 153 to 156) for the knees, hips, and back twice daily
- Ride a stationary bike to strengthen muscles supporting the knees
- Do stretching exercises to stay flexible and avoid falling
- Lose weight (see Rx #1) and stay on the Pain-Free Diet to reduce inflammation
- Take prescribed medications (talk to your physician)

Hip Pain

Hip pain is common and can be caused by osteoarthritis, bursitis, and other types of arthritis. Hip pain can also be felt when the main problem is in the spine in the lower back.

Since there are many problems that cause hip pain, some of which are serious medical problems, it is a good idea to see your doctor if the hip pain last more than 1 to 2 weeks. If your hip pain is caused by osteoarthritis, then begin the Pain-Free Diet and exercise regimen for relief of pain and long-term control.

Treatment Plan for Hip Pain

■ Apply moist heat twice daily to affected area (soak in a Jacuzzi or tub of warm water)
■ Lose weight (see Step 1) and stay on the Pain-Free Diet to reduce inflammation
■ Do range of-motion exercises (pages 153 to 156) for the hips, knees, and back
■ Swim and do water exercises to avoid added pressure on the hips
■ Monitor your stress and sleep habits using the suggestions in Rx #3 and #4
■ Take prescribed medications (talk to your doctor)

Foot Pain

Foot pain can be caused by osteoarthritis or other types of arthritis, but it can also be caused by other medical problems. If your foot pain is new or does not seem to be part of your expected arthritis pain then it is worthwhile to see your doctor to be sure no new problem is present. For example, diabetes mellitus can cause pain and other feelings in the feet and requires treatment. A second type of arthritis might be present along with osteoarthritis, and you might need several different treatments. Or you may have an undetected fracture in one of the bones of the foot.

If your foot pain is found to be due to osteoarthritis, then begin the Pain-Free Diet to reduce pressure on the foot. Exercises are important to keep the muscles strong and the joints moving in a full range of motion. Also consider seeing a podiatrist or orthopedist to be sure that you are using the most effective treatments for quick relief.

Treatment Plan for Foot Pain
- Apply moist heat twice daily to the affected area (soak in a tub or pot of warm water)
- Lose weight (see Rx #1) and stay on the Pain-Free Diet to reduce inflammation
- Do range-of-motion exercises for the feet, ankles, knees, and back
- Swim to avoid pressure on the affected area
- Take prescribed medications (talk to your physician)

Sports Injuries

Weekend activities can result in painful injuries to the back, neck, knee, shoulder, and other areas. These can happen from yard work—not only athletic events. The most common injuries are from muscle strain, bursitis, and tendinitis. These injuries are best treated with ice packs the first 2 days, and then moist heat applications twice daily until the pain has resolved. Medications to relieve pain, including the over-the-counter medications listed on pages 234 to 235, may give relief in a few days. If your pain lasts longer than a few days, check with your doctor to be sure a more serious problem is not present. In some cases, you might need an x-ray or other test to make an accurate diagnosis and get the best treatment or medication.

Treatment Plan for Sports Injuries
- Use ice packs for the first 48 hours, then apply moist heat twice daily on affected area
- Lose weight (see Rx #1) and stay on the Pain-Free Diet to reduce inflammation
- Do stretches (beginning page 162) and range-of-motion exercises (pages 153 to 159) to increase balance and muscle strength
- Avoid further injury and check with your doctor if not improved in a few days
- Select sports and recreational activities that are age appropriate

Carpal Tunnel Syndrome

In carpal tunnel syndrome, the median nerve that travels down the arm into the hand is compressed as it passes through a narrow path or tunnel at the wrist. Overuse, repetitive stress (such as computer usage or playing a musical instrument), arthritis, injury, and other problems can cause carpal tunnel syndrome. You might feel numbness, tingling, or pain in the thumb and next three fingers. The pain and numbness may travel up your arm and awaken you at night, or it may interfere with driving or holding the telephone receiver.

Your doctor can diagnose carpal tunnel syndrome with a few simple tests.

Treatment Plan for Carpal Tunnel Syndrome
- Apply moist heat twice daily to the affected areas
- Avoid the repetitive activity
- Use a splint on the affected wrist(s)
- Take a NSAID (page 235) to alleviate the pain and promote healing
- If the above result in no relief, talk to your doctor about a local injection or simple outpatient surgical procedure

Selecting
Medications

Although the goal of *Diet for a Pain-Free Life* is to help you be as active as possible with less reliance on medications, there are times when they may be necessary to help control pain and reduce inflammation. The need for medication may be temporary with an injury or sore muscle. Or with some forms of chronic arthritis, such treatment may be longer term. These drugs may allow you to do exercises and be active, which will improve your pain.

Some medications are fast acting and provide good relief for mild to moderate pain. They can be taken as needed when the pain is present, such as for a painful back or neck after a weekend of gardening or exercise. Other medications, including those for some types of rheumatoid arthritis, may take longer to work and must be taken regularly for at least a few months to have an effect.

Check with your doctor to be you are taking the best medication for your problem, with the lowest risk of side effects. Together, you can discuss the choices, including treatments you have already tried and especially any that have caused problems for you in the past. The more you know about the latest medications and their benefits and risks, the better pain control you will be able to achieve.

Be sure to follow the directions on the bottle unless your doctor tells you otherwise. If you see more than one doctor, make sure they all know about the medications you are taking to avoid unwanted drug interactions.

Over-the-Counter Pain Medications

Over-the-counter medications are used for mild to moderate pain of arthritis, neck pain, back pain, overuse, and injury. Aspirin blocks the production of prostaglandins, the chemicals in the body that trigger pain, inflammation, and swelling. Aspirin also helps reduce inflammation and pain, but in higher doses it increases the risk of serious side effects such as peptic ulcers and bleeding. Ibuprofen and naproxen are available over-the-counter in doses that have a low risk of side effects, if taken as directed. Acetaminophen elevates the pain threshold, so you perceive less pain. Acetaminophen can help ease pain with few side effects, if taken as directed on the label.

Commonly Used Over-the-Counter Pain Medications

BRAND NAME	GENERIC NAME
Advil	ibuprofen
Aleve	naproxen
Anacin	aspirin
Anacin-3	acetaminophen
Anacin Maximum Strength	acetaminophen
Ascriptin, buffered aspirin	aspirin
Bayer	aspirin
Bufferin	buffered aspirin
Excedrin Extra Strength	aspirin, acetaminophen
Motrin IB	ibuprofen
Nuprin	ibuprofen
Orudis	ketoprofen
Panex	acetaminophen
Tylenol	acetaminophin
Vanquish	aspirin, acetaminophen

Many other over-the-counter pain medications are available.

If you have abdominal pain or heartburn, stop any of these medications until you talk to your doctor. If you take blood thinners such as warfarin (Coumadin), don't take an over-the-counter pain medication without first checking with your doctor.

Prescription Nonsteroidal Anti-inflammatory Drugs (NSAIDs)

These prescription-strength medications are used when there is pain and inflammation from many types of arthritis and other pain problems. They are commonly used to treat back pain, neck pain, TMJ, injuries, headache, PMS, menstrual pain, dental pain, muscle pain, fibromyalgia, osteoarthritis, and inflammatory arthritis. These drugs work as an anti-inflammatory and pain reliever. Like aspirin, NSAIDs block the production of prostaglandins that cause inflammation, pain, and stiffness.

Commonly Used Nonsteroidal Anti-inflammatory Drugs (NSAIDs)

BRAND NAME	GENERIC NAME
Motrin	ibuprofen
Ansaid	flurbiprofen
Arthrotec	diclofenac (plus misoprostol)
Aspirin products	aspirin
Cataflam	diclofenac
Celebrex	celecoxib
Clinoril	sulindac
Daypro	oxazoprin
Disalcid, Salflex	salsalate
Dolobid	diflunisal
Feldene	piroxicam
Indocin	indomethacin
Lodine	etodolac
Magan	magnesium salicylate
Mobic	meloxicam
Naprosyn EC	naproxen (enteric-coated)

BRAND NAME	GENERIC NAME
Naprelan	naproxen
Naprosyn	naproxen
Oruvail	ketoprofen delayed release
Relafen	nabumetone
Voltaren	diclofenac

There are over twenty NSAIDs available, and one may offer relief although it may take trying several different ones to find the best results. Your doctor can guide you to the most effective one with the fewest side effects. If you develop indigestion, heartburn, abdominal pain, or swelling in the feet or legs, or your blood pressure rises, then stop the medication until you check with your doctor. Some NSAIDs, such as Celebrex (celecoxib) and Mobic (meloxicam), may have a lower risk of peptic ulcer disease and bleeding. If you have had a heart attack or stroke, or your doctor feels that you are at high risk for either, then use Celebrex with caution until further information is available concerning the possible cardiovascular risk.

If you are over sixty-five, take prednisone, or aspirin, or have had peptic ulcer disease or heart failure, you may be at higher risk for bleeding peptic ulcer. These medications should be taken with caution if you have kidney disease, hypertension, heart failure, diabetes mellitus, asthma, or lupus. These should not be taken if you are pregnant or if you take anticoagulants such as warfarin. Alcohol also increases the risk of peptic ulcers with these medications. Don't combine more than one type of NSAID unless your doctor advises it. (In most cases, it is acceptable to take a low dose of aspirin for cardiovascular protection along with the prescribed NSAID. But you might need a medication to protect from peptic ulcer and bleeding)

If you are prescribed these medications, your doctor may take blood tests to check for anemia, along with specific kidney and liver tests and other studies for safety every few months.

If you take an NSAID daily, you can protect your stomach by adding one of the protective medications listed. These can lower the risk of peptic ulcer disease and bleeding.

- Prilosec (omeprazole)
- Prevacid (lansoprazole)

- Aciphex (rabeprazole)
- Protonix (pantoprazole)
- Nexium (esomeprazole)
- Cytotec (misoporostol)

Corticosteroids

In some situations, *corticosteroids* are prescribed to treat back pain, neck pain, TMJ, carpal tunnel injuries, headache, muscle pain, osteoarthritis, inflammatory arthritis, and bone pain, among others. These medications inhibit the production of prostaglandins and leukotrienes, as well as that of certain cytokines.

Cortisone medications can help pain and swelling in arthritis and other pain conditions quickly, but with chronic use there can be many unwanted side effects, including weight gain, bone loss leading to osteoporosis, diabetes mellitus, infection, and many others. These medications can be given by tablet or injection and may be used daily, every other day, in short high-dose "bursts," or in tapered dosing.

Commonly Used Corticosteroids

BRAND NAME	GENERIC NAME
Deltasone, Sterapred	prednisone
Medrol	methylprednisolone
Prelone, Orapred	prednisolone
Decadron	dexamethasone

Stronger Medications for Pain

Narcotic pain relievers (also called opioids) are often prescribed for more intense pain or pain that does not respond to other medications. These drugs work on the central nervous system pain receptors to reduce the perception of pain. They are available in a wide variety of delivery systems, including patches and liquids, in addition to the standard dosage forms.

These stronger medications should be used carefully with your doctor's supervision but may help while other treatments take effect. Sedation, sleepiness, dizziness, and constipation can happen with the narcotic pain relievers.

If taken regularly, withdrawal symptoms may happen when stopped suddenly. Higher doses can be dangerous with respiratory depression and might warrant emergency treatment.

Commonly Used Narcotic Pain Relievers

BRAND NAME	GENERIC NAME
Darvon	propoxyphene
Darvocet, Wygesic	propoxyphene with acetaminophen
Darvon Compound	propoxyphene with aspirin
Demerol	meperidine
Duragesic (patch)	fentanyl
Kadian, MS Contin, Avenzia	morphine
Oxycontin, Oxy IR	oxycodone
Stadol (nasal spray)	butorphanol
Talwin NX	pentazocine with naloxone
Tylenol #2,3,4, Phenaphen with codeine	codeine with acetaminophen
Tylox, Percocet, Roxicet	oxycodone with acetaminophen
Vicodin, Lortab, Lorcet, Norco	hydrocodone with acetaminophen
Vicoprofen	hydrocodone with ibuprofen

Muscle Relaxants

These medications are helpful to ease painful muscle spasms and work in the central nervous system to "relax" skeletal muscles. Side effects include dry mouth, dizziness, or sleepiness. Since some drug interactions are possible, be sure your doctor is aware of other drugs you are taking when these are used.

Commonly Used Muscle Relaxants

BRAND NAME	GENERIC NAME
Flexeril	cyclobenzaprine
Kemstrol	baclofen

BRAND NAME	GENERIC NAME
Norflex	orphenadrine citrate
Parafon	chlorzoxazone
Robaxin	methocarbamol
Skelaxin	metaxalone
Soma	carisoprodol
Zanaflex	tizanidine

Adjunct Analgesics

Adjunct analgesics are medications that were originally used for other medical problems. For instance, tricyclic antidepressants were first made for treatment of depression. Over time, researchers found that if these drugs are taken in low doses, they are effective in reducing pain in fibromyalgia syndrome, neck pain, and back pain. Tricyclic antidepressants even help improve sleep in some persons. These antidepressants also increase levels of the neurotransmitters serotonin and norepinephrine in the brain. Patients with chronic pain have decreased levels of these calming neurotransmitters. Side effects of tricyclic antidepressants include drowsiness, dizziness, dry mouth, slowing of urination, and constipation, especially in older persons.

Another type of adjunct analgesics, the selective serotonin reuptake inhibitors (SSRIs), were originally developed to treat depression. Today, they are also used to treat pain, especially in fibromyalgia, back pain, neck pain and other problems. Side effects include drowsiness, sweating, nervousness, and weight gain. These medications can have some interaction with other medications so check with your doctor before you take an SSRI.

Commonly Used Tricyclic Antidepressants

BRAND NAME	GENERIC NAME
Elavil	amitriptyline
Desyrel	trazodone
Norpramin	desipramine
Pamelor	nortriptyline

BRAND NAME	GENERIC NAME
Sinequan	doxepin
Tofranil	imipramine

Commonly Used Selective Serotonin Reuptake Inhibitors

BRAND NAME	GENERIC NAME
Celexa	Citalopram
Paxil	Paroxetine
Prozac	Fluoxetine
Serzone	Nefazodone
Zoloft	Sertraline

Other medications that are increasingly used for easing pain include Cymbalta (duloxetine), a selective serotonin and norepinephrine reuptake inhibitor (SSNRI) and Lyrica (pregabalin), a medicine designed to relieve the burning, stabbing, or shooting symptoms associated with neuropathic or nerve pain. Because each person responds differently to pain medications, periodic consultations with your doctor to evaluate your pain, your medications and your overall health is necessary to stay pain free without having to deal with serious side effects.

Frequently Asked Questions

Effective communication with your doctor could save you days of suffering, especially if your pain problem has some easy solutions. At our clinic in Tampa, we find that many people wait too long before seeking an accurate diagnosis for pain. After you read this book, we encourage you to write down your questions and talk with your doctor about your concerns. Once you understand the specific cause of your pain and how it is best treated, you can take immediate measures to begin the *Diet for a Pain-Free Life*.

Also, check out our Web site at www.painfreediet.com, for continuous updates on the latest methods to resolve pain, including tips on diet, weight loss, inflammation, exercise, stress management, and sleep.

The following represent answers to questions we hear most frequently at our clinics from those who are actively seeking a cure for their pain.

Osteoarthritis, Neck, and Back Pain

Q. *I feel tired and achy most mornings. I realize that some of this might have to do with my age (79) but I'd like to know if it's normal and if I can improve it.*

A. Your aches and pains may be related to osteoarthritis, the "wear-and-tear" arthritis, which is extremely common especially in adults over age fifty. Still, check with your doctor to be sure there are no other specific problems that need to be addressed. Adding exercise to your daily activities would be a good idea if your doctor allows you to begin the exercises on pages 151 to 167. Start very gradually with 1 or 2 repetitions, then gradually increase up to 20 repetitions twice a day. This will increase the flexibility and strength of the joints and muscles, and is an important part of your Pain-Free program. Remember that it takes a few weeks for you to feel a difference in pain and stiffness. Then the longer you do the exercises, the better you'll feel. You may want to make an appointment with a physical therapist to get started on the exercises. Then you can be sure you are doing the exercises correctly to get full benefit.

Along with exercise, Prescription #1, the Pain-Free Diet, can give you exceptional relief of inflammation and pain. Follow the guidelines beginning on page 31. If any specific foods trigger more pain (such as tomato products), avoid these foods for more relief. Some medications may be helpful during times of more pain and stiffness, or before you do exercises. If your doctor says that you can use over-the-counter pain medications, try acetaminophen, ibuprofen, or naproxen. If you get no relief and the pain still limits your ability to be active, then talk to your doctor about the problem and see if a prescription pain medication might help. This may include a mild pain reliever that can be used only as needed.

Q. *My orthopedist recommended that I try a TENS unit for my lower back pain. How does this work?*

A. Transcutaneous electrical nerve stimulation (TENS) is a pain treatment that uses small amounts of electrical stimulation to help block the nerve signals that carry pain messages to the spinal cord and brain. Electrode pads are placed in proper areas, depending on your pain location, with a small battery pack that is often worn on the belt like a pager or cell phone. The amount of electrical stimulation can be adjusted. TENS does not work for every patient but many people find that it brings some relief. You will not know if it can work for you until you try it.

Q. *I live with chronic neck and shoulder pain. I take the prescribed medications and try to exercise but the pain is often unbearable. My husband says the pain is "in my head." Do women experience more pain than men?*

A. First, it's important to know that pain is not in your head! Just because pain cannot be seen or proven with a laboratory test does not mean it is fabricated. If your husband (or anyone) doubts your pain, talk to your doctor together and let him or her explain the pain problem.

There is some new information that women may actually feel pain more often, or it may feel more severe with aging. Researchers have found that women may interpret pain in a different way and that the additional anxiety that accompanies pain may affect how women interpret the overall pain. This doesn't change how pain is treated. But it does indicate that everyone with pain should be aware of corresponding problems, such as anxiety, insomnia, or depression, which can be specifically treated to give even better improvement in alleviating the pain and discomfort.

Q. *I've tried moist heat, and it does not help my neck pain. What else can I use?*

A. If heat doesn't work, try cold therapy. Use ice or cold packs but *never* apply ice directly to your skin, or you might experience more than neck pain! You might also try a local spray such as fluromethane (nonflammable) on your neck or another painful area before and after exercise. This superficial cooling decreases muscle spasms and increases the pain threshold. Some patients prefer cold therapy to moist heat for acute pain, while others tell of having the best relief when they alternate the sessions with moist heat and ice. I suggest that you choose the method of moist heat and ice packs that gives the best relief with the least trouble or expense. (Again, always use caution to avoid damage to your skin with hot and cold therapies.)

Q. *My colleague sees a physician who uses acupressure and acupuncture to treat low back pain. Can this really work?*

A. *Acupuncture* is thousands of years old and can be used for many types of pain. It is an accepted complementary treatment for arthritis, back pain, fibromyalgia, and many other types of chronic pain. Objective trials show a response in many cases and when there is a response it is often dramatic. However, it may be a little hard to predict which person will respond. Overall, I believe that it should be considered as a possibility if the person is already following the Pain-Free Diet, along with stress management, daily exercises, sleep strategies, and medication. Quite honestly, you will not know whether acupressure or acupuncture works for you until you try it. I do suggest that you choose a qualified acupuncturist, and do not hesitate to ask about that person's experience and training.

Q. *I sit at the computer for most of the day. When I finally get up to go home, my back is so stiff I feel a hundred years old. What can I do to prevent this?*

A. Even with no arthritis problems, many who sit at their computer all day notice pain and stiffness. The best prevention is exercise, especially movements that keep the muscles of the neck, back and shoulders strong and flexible. Diet and weight control are also important, which is why the Pain-Free Diet has helped many of my patients overcome work-related pain and stiffness. Taking a very short break, even walking around your desk every 15 minutes, can help prevent stiffness.

It's important to make sure that your computer workstation fits you. Studies show that in businesses or organizations where workstation furniture is not adjustable or ergonomically correct, it can result in on-the-job-pain and stiffness in more than one-third of workers. Many times people have chairs that lack adequate back support, and workers often assumed positions that were not recommended in an attempt to avoid pain.

Try to avoid having a fixed posture and make sure your seat has good lumbar support. Also, prolonged sitting and inactivity can increase back pain and lead to disk degeneration. Strive for better muscle function with daily exercise. Also, avoid fixed postures and chairs without good lumbar support to prevent further back problems.

Q. *I work for hours at my computer desk at work. What can I do to alleviate the muscle tension and pain in my lower back?*

A. Strong muscles in the lower back and pelvis are crucial to keep proper body alignment while sitting. When you slump while sitting, those muscles are less active and therefore give less support. Sitting leads to inactivity, which can result in disk degeneration and disk herniation.

To keep your back supported while sitting, use a lumbar disk support. You can roll up a thick bath towel and put this behind your waist when sitting at your desk. Or you can buy a lumbar support at a medical supply store. Also, sit on a foam cushion to protect your tailbone from injury and pain. You can cut a piece of foam the size of the seat of your chair, and then cut a 4-inch circle out of the center to relieve pressure. Or you can buy a ready-made "doughnut" cushion at most medical supply stores or pharmacies.

Equally important is to select an ergonomically correct chair with strong back support. Sitting with no back support increases the force on the spine by about 40 percent more than does standing. Leaning forward when you sit causes even higher forces. A reclined posture with your chair back at a slight angle often works best to keep you pain free. When you sit in the chair, your buttocks should press against the back of the chair. Your feet should be flat on the floor. Your knees should be slightly higher than your hips, and you shouldn't have to strain to see your computer. Use a footstool, if possible, to ease pressure off your back. Make sure your chair has an armrest, as it helps to take some of the strain off your neck and shoulders.

It's also important to get up from your chair and move around for several minutes every 15 to 30 minutes. Do some of the stretches listed on pages 163 to 165 to loosen tight joints, ligaments, muscles, and tendons.

Fibromyalgia Syndrome

Q. *After years of living with deep muscle pain, I finally got the diagnosis of fibromyalgia syndrome. What causes this problem?*

A. The cause of fibromyalgia is not known. Some patients get fibromyalgia after an accident or after surgery, whereas others simply develop the problem without any apparent reason. Most report being highly sensitive to pain, fatigue, and poor sleep habits. Here are some of the possible contributing causes of fibromyalgia:

- Aging
- Decrease in serotonin (a chemical in the body often associated with calming and antianxiety)
- Female gender
- High sensitivity to pain (even from normally nonpainful stimulation)
- Inherited tendency

- Injury to the nervous system
- Magnesium deficiency
- Menopause
- Poor physical conditioning
- Result of depression
- Result of injury or accident
- Side effect of flu
- Sleep disorder
- Stress
- Surgery

Review the information on page 224 and follow the suggested treatment plan, which includes twice-daily applications of moist heat, exercises, stretching, and managing stress and sleep habits. Also talk to your doctor about medication, if needed. Some people are finding that a low-dose antidepressant helps patients with fibromyalgia increase the quality of their sleep and reduces pain.

Bursitis

Q. *I continue to have bursitis in my left hip, especially after sitting for lengthy periods or bending over doing yard work. What causes this?*

A. There are many different causes of bursitis, but the most common type is caused by wear-and-tear changes and repetitive movements of the muscles and tendons as they slide through the bursa sac. For example, bursitis in the shoulder can happen after overdoing your activities around the house on the weekend. This can make it very painful just to lift your arm above your shoulder. An injury can also cause inflammation of the area and pain on movement. Your doctor can make sure no other causes, such as infection, are present that need specific treatment. If it is just bursitis, one of the medications on page 234 may be prescribed along with moist heat and rest, then gradually increasing the functional fitness exercises of Rx #3.

Q. *If you lift your arm up and down and feel a little "pop" is that abnormal? What if you are stretching and you feel a little pop in your upper back? Are these signs of arthritis even if there is no pain?*

A. The pop you feel may be from a tendon as it moves over the shoulder and, unless it is painful and persistent, it is not usually a sign of a serious problem. The sensation felt in the back muscles may be from excessive stretching of a muscle. It might cause some soreness later especially if there is a muscle strain. Some people do this stretching deliberately. A good warm-up, using the functional fitness exercises in Rx #3 can usually prevent serious muscle strain.

If the knee is painful and pops when it moves or if it locks in one position, it could be a sign of a problem in a ligament or cartilage in the knee. A small piece of cartilage (called a loose body) may cause the knee to lock and make it very hard or painful to move for a few minutes. If you have persistent pain or locking or weakness in a knee, it is best to check it out with your doctor.

Carpal Tunnel Syndrome

Q. *I am a technical writer and have noticed tingling and numbness in my right wrist. Are these symptoms of carpal tunnel? If so, how should this be treated?*

A. The symptoms of carpal tunnel syndrome include pain and tingling or numbness in the thumb and next three fingers, with the exception of the little finger. You may also feel swelling in your fingers. Sometimes there may be pain that travels from the hand up the arm, possibly to the elbow.

The pain, numbness, and tingling usually worsen at night and while driving or holding the telephone. Some claim the symptoms increase when the hand is warm and decrease when it is cool. You may even wake up with your hand(s) asleep and have to shake it to try to regain feeling.

As carpal tunnel syndrome progresses, your hand may become noticeably weaker so that daily activities such as opening a jar or grasping your hairbrush may be difficult. You may drop items easily and think you're just plain clumsy—when, in fact, the CTS has weakened your grip.

Depending on the exact cause, treatment may include one of the medications listed on page 235, along with a splint for your wrist, and a local injection of cortisone to reduce the swelling around the nerve. A surgical procedure can be planned by your doctor for relief. The Pain-Free Diet will help reduce pro-inflammatory markers in the body, which can help ease pain. The exercise suggestions on page 157 are also important, as you take frequent breaks from the computer and focus on stretching the arm and wrist.

Rheumatoid Arthritis

Q. *I've had rheumatoid arthritis for almost a decade. Are there any new medications available that have fewer serious side effects? What recommendations would you give someone with rheumatoid?*

A. The treatment for rheumatoid arthritis has improved dramatically—so much that arthritis specialists now believe that every patient has a chance of complete control of pain and swelling. You should have two goals with rheumatoid arthritis: (1) control of the pain, swelling and stiffness; and (2) control of long-term damage to the joints to prevent deformity. These two goals can almost always be achieved with the available treatments.

The combination of treatments that work best include the Pain-Free Diet, stress management, daily exercise and movement, quality sleep, and the most effective anti-inflammatory medication and suppressive medications to control the inflammation and prevent joint damage. Because about 70 percent of rheumatoid arthritis patients are at risk for long-term joint damage, which can cause deformity and loss of use of the joints, it is important to start treatment early. The suppressive medications help turn off the process that causes inflammation and joint damage.

The suppressive treatments, including methotrexate (Trexall, Rheumatrex) and leflunamide (Arava), which are usually given in pill form, help 70 to 80 percent of patients when the best dose is achieved. If the above two goals are still not met, then many patients may benefit from one of the newer biologic medications. These revolutionary medications are injected by the patient at home or are given by intravenous injection in the clinic. These biologic medications often give dramatic improvement in pain, swelling, stiffness, and fatigue. They also can stop the joint damage and destruction.

There are some potential side effects with the biologic medications, including the possibility of infections, but these can be managed by your arthritis specialist. You have to consider the benefits compared to the risks for each treatment. More drugs than ever are available, so it is more likely than ever that you can find the one that gives you relief without side effects. Above all else, early treatment is the key.

Biologic Medications for Inflammatory Arthritis

- Humira
- Enbrel
- Remicade
- Kineret
- Orencia
- Rituxin

Foot Pain

Q. *After a longer period of working in the yard or walking the stairs at work, I have a pain in the heel area on the bottom of my feet. The pain is exaggerated if I am not wearing shoes, but seems to lessen when I wear shoes. I love to walk and work in my yard. What can I do to avoid this painful condition?*

A. The pain in the middle of the heel on the bottom of your foot is most often due to a problem called plantar fasciitis, which is caused by inflammation of the tissues that attach at the bottom of the heel. It will hurt when you walk as the heel touches the ground, so every step may be painful. If your doctor confirms this, it usually helps to soak the heel or foot in warm water twice a day for 15 to 20 minutes, and to buy a good heel cushion at your sporting goods store or pharmacy. Use the heel cushion in your shoe or sock anytime you're up during the day. If your pain continues, a local injection or other medications from your doctor can help. This problem usually will take care of itself over a few weeks.

The Pain-Free Diet

Q. *I reviewed the Pain-Free Diet, but I cannot eat just fruits and vegetables. Why is beef or pork not allowed on your program?*

A. Animal foods contribute to inflammation by increasing the body's supply of pro-inflammatory chemicals, as discussed on page 33. When animal foods are replaced with fish, low-fat dairy products, and plant protein, the body creates less inflammation, resulting in less pain. If omega-3 fatty acids and others anti-inflammatory supplements are also added to the diet, they further decrease inflammation and pain. The main outcome of the Pain-Free Diet is that people on the regimen feel full and lose weight, particularly waistline or belly fat, which is known to also increase pro-inflammatory markers and increase the risk of serious illness such as cardiovascular disease and diabetes.

Surgery

Q. *How do I know if I need surgery on my arthritic hip? I have pain all the time and even medications don't give me relief. What types of surgery are available and are they safe?*

A. If you do not find enough relief from pain and inflammation using medications, exercise, and moist heat applications, then your doctor may suggest surgery as a last resort to eliminate pain and allow you to be active. Especially when your pain is constant and severe or the joint has become very limited by arthritis despite treatment, surgery is a viable treatment alternative. For example, in osteoarthritis, the cartilage of the knee or hip may be so damaged that no medication will help. Or, in rheumatoid arthritis, there may be so much swelling and thickening of the joint lining that medications may not be effective.

While I prefer my patients to try nonsurgical treatments, including the four prescriptions in this program, joint replacement surgery does relieve pain and may allow you to return to a more normal activity level. Sometimes joint surgery may eliminate the pain and limitation of arthritis. This can change severe limitation and loss of independence to independent living again.

To decide if you are a good candidate for joint replacement surgery, you must consider the level of pain you feel and how it has affected your quality of life. I always tell my patients that if their pain is constant and incapacitating, and if activity or exercise is limited even after weight loss, regular exercise, and good medical treatment, then surgery may be a consideration. A question I always ask patients to consider is: "What if you had *no* pain in the knee (or hip or shoulder)?" If your quality of life, including exercise and pain level, would be excellent with less pain, then surgery might be beneficial.

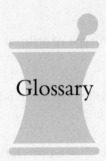

Glossary

Activities of daily living (ADLs): The activities we normally do in daily living including feeding ourselves, bathing, dressing, grooming, work, homemaking, and leisure.

Acupuncture: The practice of putting needles into the body for health benefits, such as to reduce pain.

Aerobic exercise: Any exercise that promotes the oxygen circulation in the blood (running, cycling, swimming, and in-line skating).

Allergen: A substance such as pollen, mold, or animal dander that may produce an allergic reaction.

Alternative therapies: Healing techniques that are not usually scientific in nature nor generally taught in medical schools.

Antinuclear antibodies (ANAs): ANAs are found in some patients whose immune system is prone to cause inflammation against their own body tissues. They are found in patients with a number of autoimmune diseases, such as systemic lupus erythematosus, Sjogren's syndrome, rheumatoid arthritis, polymyositis, and scleroderma, among others.

Analgesic: Analgesics are medications that relieve pain. Some are over-the-counter, some require a doctor's prescription. Over-the-counter analgesics are nonnarcotic. Analgesics available by prescription can be narcotic or nonnarcotic. There are other medications that function as analgesics but were developed for other purposes. These medications are often referred to as "adjunctive pain relievers."

Ankylosing spondylitis: A type of arthritis that causes chronic inflammation of the spine.

Antigen: Something potentially capable of inducing an immune response. Antigens elicit antibodies.

Anti-inflammatory: Agents that reduce inflammation without directly antagonizing the agent that caused it.

Apheresis: A technique in which blood is taken, treated or separated, then returned to the donor.

Arachidonic acid: A fatty acid that is converted to pro-inflammatory chemicals, which lead to disease, inflammation, and increased pain.

Arteritis, temporal: This serious inflammatory disease of the arteries is also called "giant cell arteritis" or "cranial arteritis," and is more common after age fifty. It is detected by a biopsy of an artery and is treated with cortisone. If left untreated, it can lead to blindness or stroke.

Arthritis: Inflammation of a joint that can develop into swelling, stiffness, warmth, redness, and pain. There are more than one hundred types of arthritis, including osteoarthritis, rheumatoid arthritis, ankylosing spondylitis, psoriatic arthritis, lupus, gout, and pseudogout, among others.

Arthritis, rheumatoid: An autoimmune disease characterized by chronic inflammation of the joints and can cause inflammation of tissues in other areas of the body (such as the lungs, heart, and eyes).

Back pain, low: Pain in the lower back that may come from the bony lumbar spine, disks between the vertebrae, ligaments around the spine and disks, spinal cord and nerves, muscles of the low back, internal organs of the pelvis and abdomen, and the skin covering the lumbar area.

Body mass index (BMI): BMI calculates weight compared to height. Those with a higher per cent body fat tend to have a higher BMI than those who have a greater per cent of muscle.

BMI 18.5 or less	Underweight
BMI 18.6 to 24.9	Acceptable weight
BMI 25 to 29.9	Overweight
BMI 30 and higher	Obese

Bone scan: A test which is done to detect abnormal areas of bone from such problems as fracture, infection, or cancer.

Bursitis: A bursa is a closed fluid-filled sac that functions as a gliding surface to reduce friction between tissues of the body. When the bursa becomes inflamed, the condition is known as "bursitis."

C-reactive protein (CRP): A protein normally made by the body that can be measured in the blood as one index of inflammation. The body increases the production of C-reactive protein with infections or inflammation of many types. In such problems as arthritis, the level of CRP is increased when the arthritis is active, and lower as the arthritis improves. Some studies have shown that a higher level of CRP can be associated with higher risk of cardiovascular disease, heart attack, and diabetes.

Calcium: A mineral in the body found mainly in the hard part of bones. Calcium is essential for healthy bones, as well as for muscle contraction, heart action, and normal blood clotting. Food sources of calcium include dairy foods, most dark leafy green vegetables such as broccoli and collards, canned salmon, clams, oysters, calcium-fortified foods, and tofu.

Carpal tunnel syndrome: A problem that causes numbness or tingling in the hand, especially on the palm side, and mainly around the thumb and next three fingers in some combination. There are many causes, including work-related from computer use and arthritis. Treatment is available for symptoms, including wearing a splint, local injection, and surgery to correct it.

Cartilage: Firm, rubbery tissue that cushions bones at joints.

Childhood arthritis: Arthritis that happens before age sixteen is called "juvenile arthritis." Almost 50 percent of these cases have a chance of spontaneous remission or disappearance of the symptoms at any age during childhood or adolescence.

Chronic: An illness or problem that lasts a long time, usually three months or more.

Clinical trials: Medical research studies conducted by government or private industry. Usually, volunteers are recruited into "control groups" in which experimental treatments for the detection, prevention, or cure of medical conditions are applied.

Corticosteroid: Any of the steroid hormones made by the cortex (outer layer) of the adrenal gland. Cortisol is a corticosteroid.

Cortisol: One of several types of hormones produced by the body which is commonly associated with stress and acute illnesses.

COX-1: One of two types of COX enzyme, it causes the production of the prostaglandins which help protect the stomach and other organs.

COX-2: The other type of COX enzyme, it causes the production of the prostaglandins that create inflammation pain and may be involved in some cancers, such as colon cancer, and Alzheimer's disease.

Cytokine: One of the proteins the body makes in inflammation to fight infection and other diseases. When cytokines are overproduced they can cause damage to the body itself. In rheumatoid arthritis, increased production of cytokines cause joint pain, swelling, stiffness, fatigue, and permanent joint damage.

Degenerative arthritis: *see* Osteoarthritis

Degenerative joint disease: *see* Osteoarthritis

Fibromyalgia syndrome: Fibromyalgia syndrome causes chronic deep muscle pain, stiffness, and tenderness without detectable inflammation. Fibromyalgia does not cause body damage or deformity. However, undue fatigue plagues 90 percent of patients.

Gout: An arthritic condition characterized by abnormally elevated levels of uric acid in the blood, recurring attacks of joint inflammation (arthritis), deposits of hard lumps of uric acid in and around the joints, and decreased kidney function and kidney stones. The tendency to develop gout and elevated blood uric acid level (hyperuricemia) is often inherited and can be promoted by obesity, weight gain, alcohol intake, high blood pressure, abnormal kidney function, and drugs.

Inflammation: Localized redness, warmth, swelling and pain because of infection, irritation, or injury.

Immune response: Any response by the immune system.

Internal medicine: A medical specialty dedicated to the diagnosis and medical treatment of adults. A physician who specializes in internal medicine is called an "internist." A minimum of seven years of medical school and postgraduate training are focused on learning the prevention, diagnosis, and treatment of diseases of adults.

Lumbar stenosis: A narrowing of the lower part of the spine, which causes pressure on the spinal nerves. Lumbar stenosis usually causes lower back pain; it is often worse when walking and is then relieved by resting a few minutes. The pain can travel down the legs and may gradually worsen. It can be treated with medications and/or surgery.

Lupus: *see* SLE

Nonsteroid anti-inflammatory drugs (NSAIDS): Standard medications for the treatment of arthritis; they decrease inflammation and pain by reducing the enzyme cyclooxygenase (COX). COX creates inflammation molecules in the body. The older COX-1 medicines (aspirin, ibuprofen, naproxen) have a higher risk of peptic ulcer and bleeding if used alone. The

COX-2 medicines have a lower risk of peptic ulcers and bleeding but some have been associated with a possible higher risk of heart attack and stroke in some patients. Both COX-1 and COX-2 NSAIDs work to reduce inflammation.

Nodule: A small collection of tissue. The word *nodule* is the diminutive of *node* (a knot or knob) so a *nodule* means "a little knot or knob."

Obstructive sleep apnea (OSA): A disorder where people literally stop breathing repeatedly during their sleep.

Orthopedics: The branch of surgery broadly concerned with the skeletal system (bones).

Osteoarthritis: Type of arthritis caused by breakdown, and eventual loss of the cartilage of the joints (also called "degenerative arthritis" or "degenerative joint disease").

Osteoporosis: Thinning of the bones with reduction in bone mass predisposing to fractures.

Over-the-counter (OTC) medication: Any drug that may be purchased without a doctor's prescription.

Oxygen free radical: One of the chemicals produced in the body that can cause damage to cells.

Polymalgia rheumatica: A type of arthritis that causes severe pain around the shoulders, upper arms, hips, and thighs, with severe stiffness in the morning, awakening at night, and overall miserable feeling. Some patients with polymyalgia rheumatica may also have headache and temporal arteritis, inflammation in arteries, which can be dangerous and needs medical treatment quickly.

Primary care: The "medical home" for a patient, ideally providing continuity and integration of health care. All family physicians and most pediatricians and internists are in primary care.

Prostaglandin: One of several proteins in the body that can contribute to inflammation and pain in arthritis. Other prostaglandins are beneficial and help to protect the stomach and other organs.

Psoriatic arthritis: A potentially destructive and deforming form of arthritis that affects approximately 10 percent of persons with psoriasis.

Phytochemicals: The biologically active substances that give plants their deep colors, flavors, odors, and protection against disease.

Rheumatoid arthritis: An autoimmune disease, often called a "systemic" illness, which causes chronic inflammation of the joints, the tissue around the joints, as well as other organs in the body.

Rheumatoid factor: An antibody that is measurable in the blood. It is commonly used as a blood test to help in the diagnosis of rheumatoid arthritis. Rheumatoid factor is present in about 80 percent of adults

Rheumatoid nodules: Lumps that develop in Rheumatoid Arthritis over joint areas that receive pressure, such as knuckles of the hand.

Rheumatologist: An internist who specializes in arthritis and related diseases of the joints, muscles, and bones.

Ruptured disk: The cartilage disc between two vertebral bones in the spine may degenerate or be injured, and the contents of the disk may bulge backward to press on a nerve from the spinal cord. This can cause pain in the back, which often travels down a leg. The most common sites of a ruptured disk are in the lower lumbar part of the spine.

Scleroderma: A type of arthritis that causes joint pain with skin tightening, which can happen over the hands, arms, face, and other areas. It can cause internal organ disease, including esophageal and swallowing problems, hypertension, kidney disease, or lung disease.

Synovial fluid: The slippery fluid in joints, which normally nourishes the joints.

Systemic lupus erythematosus (SLE or lupus): An inflammatory disease of connective tissue occurring predominantly in women (90 percent). It is considered an autoimmune disease and is a type of arthritis that can cause joint pain and rashes, and has the potential for serious internal organ disease, such as kidney disease. SLE can affect most organs and can be life-threatening without medical treatment.

Tendinitis: An inflammation of a tendon, which attaches a muscle to a bone. It can be caused by repetitive or overuse of a muscle, such as tendinitis in an elbow or shoulder.

Trigger point: Localized areas of tenderness in muscles and other soft tissues around joints (not joints themselves) that hurt to touch.

Tumor necrosis factor (TNF): A protein produced in the body that is responsible for triggering inflammation in the joints, including pain, swelling, and causes fatigue and joint destruction in rheumatoid arthritis.

Vasculitis: An inflammation in blood vessels, which can include arteries and veins. Inflammation in arteries can cause blockage of the artery and disease in the organ the artery supplies, such as kidney disease, stroke, rash, and many other serious medical problems. There are many different specific causes of vasculitis, which can be life-threatening without treatment.

References and
Supporting Research

R. Melzack, P. D. Wall, "Pain Mechanisms: A New Theory," *Science* 150 (1965): 971.

National Center for Health Statistics. *Third National Health and Nutrition Examination Survey 1988–1994* (Atlanta, GA: Centers for Disease Control and Prevention, 1996).

P. Trayhurn and I. S. Wood, "Adipokines: Inflammation and the Pleiotropic Role of White Adipose Tissue," *British Journal of Nutrition* 92 (2004): 347–55.

M. Sharif, C. J. Elson, P. A. Dieppe, and J. Kirwan, "Elevated Serum C-Reactive Protein Levels in Osteoarthritis," *British Journal of Rheumatology* 36 (1997): 140–41.

K. Esposito, R. Marfella, M. Ciotola, et al., "Effect of a Mediterranean-Style Diet on Endothelial Dysfunction and Markers of Vascular Inflammation in the Metabolic Syndrome: A Randomized Trial, *Journal of the American Medical Association* 292, no. 12 (September 22, 2004): 1440–46.

G. Sesmilo, B. M. Biller, J. Llevadot, et al., "Effects of Growth Hormone Administration on Inflammatory and Other Cardiovascular Risk Markers in Men with Growth Hormone Deficiency: A Randomized, Controlled Clinical Trial." *Annals of Internal Medicine* 133 (2000): 111.

P. Ziccardi, F. Nappo, G. Giugliano, et al., "Reduction of Inflammatory Cytokine Concentrations and Improvement of Endothelial Functions in Obese Women after Weight Loss over One Year," *Circulation* 105 (2002): 804.

S. E. Berkow and N. Barnard, "Vegetarian Diets and Weight Status," *Nutrition Reviews* 64 (2006): 1–11.

D. S. Ludwig, M. A. Pereira, C. H. Kroenke, et al., Dietary Fiber Weight Gain, and Cardiovascular Disease Risk Factors in Young Adults," *Journal of the American Medical Association* 282 (1999): 1539.

R. Martin, I. Villegas, C. La Casa, and C. A. de la Lastra, "Resveratrol, a Polyphenol Found in Grapes, Suppresses Oxidative Damage and Stimulates Apoptosis during Early Colonic Inflammation in Rats," *Biochemical Pharmacology.* 67, no. 7 (2004): 1399–410.

E. Middleton Jr., C. Kandaswami, T. C. Theoharides, "The Effects of Plant Flavonoids on Mammalian Cells: Implications for Inflammation, Heart Disease, and Cancer," *Pharmacological Reviews* 52 (2000): 673–751.

Nature (Eberhardt, MV) 405 (2000): 903–04.

F. C. Stintzing, A. S. Stintzing, R. Carle, B. Frei, and R. E. Wrolstad, "Color and Antioxidant Properties of Cyanidin-Based Anthocyanin Pigments," *Journal of Agriccuture and Food and Chemistry.* 50, no. 21 (2002): 6172–81.

M. F. McCarty, "Low-Insulin-Response Diets May Decrease Plasma C-Reactive Protein by Influencing Adipocyte Function," *Medical Hypotheses* 64, no. 2 (2005): 385–87.

S. Liu, "Intake of Refined Carbohydrates and Whole Grain Foods in Relation to Risk of Type 2 Diabetes Mellitus and Coronary Heart Disease," *Journal of the American College of Nutrition* 21 (2002): 298.

R. S. Panush, ed., "Nutrition and Rheumatic Diseases," *Rheumatic Diseases Clinics of North America* 17 (1991): 197.

L. Bu, K. D. Setchell, and E. D. Lephart, "Influences of Dietary Soy Isoflavones on Metabolism but Not Nociception and Stress Hormone Responses in Ovariectomized Female Rats," *Reproductive Biology and Endocrinology.* (October 26, 2005): 3.

C. K. Roberts, D. Won, S. Pruthi, et al., "Effect of a short-term diet and exercise intervention on oxidative stress, inflammation, MMP-9, and monocyte chemotactic activity in men with metabolic syndrome factors," *Journal of Applied Physiology,* no. 5 (May 2006): 1657–65. E-published December 15, 2005

T. Toda, N. Segal, "Lean Body Mass and Body Fat Distribution in Participants with Chronic Low Back Pain," *Archives of Internal Medicine* 160 (2000): 3265–69.

T. S. Han, J. S. Schouten, M. E. Lean, J. C. Seidell. "The Prevalence of Low Back Pain and Associations with Body Fatness, Fat Distribution and Height," *International Journal of Obesity and Related Metabolic Disorders* 21, no. 7 (July 1997): 600–07.

B. K. McFarlin, M. G. Flynn, W. W. Campbell, B. A. Craig, J. P. Robinson, et al., "Physical Activity Status, but Not Age, Influences Inflammatory Biomarkers and Toll-Like Receptor," *Journal of Gerontology Series A Biological Sciences and Medical Science.* 61, no. 4 (April 2006): 388–93.

E. M. Lewiecki, "Management of Osteoporosis," *Clinical Molecular Allergy* 2, no. 1 (July 14, 2004): 9.

E. C. Suarez, "C-Reactive Protein Is Associated with Psychological Risk Factors of Cardiovascular Disease in Apparently Healthy Adults," *Psychosomatic Medicine,* 66, no. 5 (September/October 2004): 684–91.

G. Grossi, A. Perski, B. Evengard, V. Blomkvist, and K. Orth-Gomer, "Physiological Correlates of Burnout among Women," *Journal of Psychosomatic Research* 55, no. 4 (October 2003): 309–16.

G. B. Stefano and G. J. Dobos, "Rapid Stress Reduction and Anxiolysis Among Distressed Women as a Consequence of a Three-Month Intensive Yoga Program," *Medical Science Monitor* 11, no. 12 (December 2005): CR555–61. E-published November 24, 2005.

K. J. Sherman, D. C. Cerkin, J. Erro, et al., "Comparing Yoga, Exercise, and a Self-Care Book for Chronic Low Back Pain: A Randomized, Controlled Trial," *Annals of Internal Medicine* 143, no. 12 (December 20, 2005): 849–56.

M. Dash and S. Telles, "Improvement in Hand Grip Strength in Normal Volunteers and Rheumatoid Arthritis Patients following Yoga Training," *Indian Journal of Physiology and Pharmacology.* 45, no. 3 (July 2001): 355–60.

E. Schrader, "Equivalence of a St. John's Wort Extract (Ze 117) and Fluoxetine: A Randomized, Controlled Study in Mild-Moderate Depression," *International Clinical Psychopharmacology* 15, no. 2 (2000): 61–68.

M. Cohen-Zion and S. Ancoli-Israel. "Sleep Disorders," in W. R. Hazzard, J. P. Blass, J. B. Halter, et al., *Principles of Geriatric Medicine and Gerontology*, 5th ed. (New York: McGraw-Hill, Inc, 2003), 1531–41.

K. Krauchi, C. Cajochen, and A. Wirz-Justice, "Thermophysiologic Aspects of the Three-Process-Model of Sleepiness Regulation," *Clinics in Sports Medicine* 24, no. 2 (April 2005): ix, 287–300.

J. Herrera, M. Nava, F. Romero, et al., "Melatonin Prevents Oxidative Stress Resulting from Iron and Erythropoietin Administration," *American Journal of Kidney Diseases* 37 (2001): 750.

M. Karasek and R. J. Reiter, "Melatonin and Aging," review, in *Neuro Endocrinology Letters* 23, Suppl. 1 (2002): 14–16.

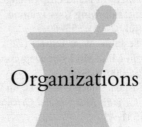

Organizations

AMERICAN DIETETIC ASSOCIATION
120 South Riverside Plaza, Suite 2000
Chicago, Illinois 60606-6995
800-877-1600
www.eatright.org/cps/rde/xchg/ada/hs.xsl/index.html

AMERICAN ACADEMY OF MEDICAL ACUPUNCTURE (AAMA)
4929 Wilshire Boulevard
Suite 428
Los Angeles, California 90010
323-937-5514
www.medicalacupuncture.org/

AMERICAN ACADEMY OF PAIN MANAGEMENT
13947 Mono Way #A
Sonora, CA 95370
209-533-9744
www.aapainmanage.org/

AMERICAN CHRONIC PAIN ASSOCIATION
P.O. Box 850
Rocklin, CA 95677
800-533-3231
www.theacpa.org/

AMERICAN COLLEGE OF RHEUMATOLOGY
1800 Century Place, Suite 250
Atlanta, GA 30345-4300
404-633-3777
www.rheumatology.org/

AMERICAN FIBROMYALGIA SYNDROME
  ASSOCIATION, INC.
6380 E. Tanque Verde, Suite D
Tucson, AZ 85715
www.afsafund.org/

AMERICAN OBESITY ASSOCIATION
1250 24th Street, NW, Suite 300
Washington, DC 20037
www.obesity.org/

AMERICAN PAIN FOUNDATION
201 N. Charles Street, Suite 710
Baltimore, Maryland 21201-4111
888-615-PAIN (7246)
www.painfoundation.org/

AMERICAN PAIN SOCIETY
4700 W. Lake Ave.
Glenview, IL 60025
847-375-4715
www.ampainsoc.org/

ARTHRITIS FOUNDATION
P.O. Box 7669
Atlanta, GA 30357-0667
Main Number: 404-872-7100
404-965-7888
800-568-4045
www.arthritis.org/

**NATIONAL CENTER FOR COMPLEMENTARY
AND ALTERNATIVE MEDICINE (NCCAM)**
9000 Rockville Pike
Bethesda, MD 20892
E-mail: info@nccam.nih.gov
http://nccam.nih.gov/

NORTH AMERICAN SPINE SOCIETY
22 Calendar Court, 2nd Floor
LaGrange, IL USA 60525
877-774-6337
www.spine.org/

SPONDYLITIS ASSOCIATION OF AMERICA
P O Box 5872
Sherman Oaks, CA 91413
800-777-8189 (U.S. only)
www.spondylitis.org/

THE ARTHRITIS SOCIETY (CANADIAN NATIONAL OFFICE)
393 University Avenue, Suite 1700
Toronto, Ontario
Canada
M5G 1E6
416-979-7228
www.arthritis.ca/custom%20home/default.asp?s=1

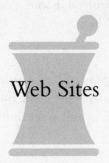

Web Sites

ADAM.COM—MEDLINE PLUS MEDICAL ENCYCLOPEDIA
ADAM.com is a leading online provider of health, medical, and wellness
information. The Medical Encyclopedia has been licensed by MEDLINE-
Plus. At this site, after choosing a topic, you can link through to an
overview, a list of symptoms, treatments, and prevention.
www.nlm.nih.gov/medlineplus/encyclopedia.html

ABLEDATA
AbleData is a great source for assistive technology information.

ACTIVE-FOREVER.COM
Active-Forever.com offers a variety of daily living aids.
www.activeforever.com

AIDS FOR ARTHRITIS (ASSISTIVE DEVICES FOR ARTHRITIS SUFFERERS)
www.aidsforarthritis.com

DYNAMIC-LIVING.COM
Dynamic-Living.com offers kitchen products, bathroom helpers, and
unique daily living aids.
www.dynamic-living.com/index.html

IMMUNESUPPORT.COM

ImmuneSupport.com is a great site, with current information on fibromyalgia and chronic fatigue syndrome.
immunesupport.com

MAYO CLINIC

Developed and reviewed by Mayo Clinic physicians and scientists, this site hosts a wealth of evidence-based, up-to-date information on various health and disease conditions, as well as specific "conditions centers."
www.mayohealth.org

MEDICINENET.COM

MedicineNet.com seeks to provide relevant, easy-to-read, in-depth medical information for consumers.
www.medicinenet.com/script/main/hp.asp

NEW YORK ONLINE ACCESS TO HEALTH (NOAH)

NOAH is a unique collection of state, local, and federal resources selected by editors and consumers in mind. Searchers may select from a list of health topics that are then narrowed to include definitions, care and treatment, and lists of information resources. NOAH has many bilingual resources, including a Spanish list of references.
www.noah-health.org/

THE KEYLESS ERGONOMIC KEYBOARDS

This site offers a keyless ergonomic keyboard solution that removes the barrier posed by the traditional keyboard/mouse combination. Persons who benefit include those with repetitive stress injuries, limited fine motor skills, reduced finger function, and other physical challenges.
www.keybowl.com/kb/index?page=home

Acknowledgments

IN OUR QUEST to give accurate and up-to-date information on pain problems and the breakthrough information on diet and inflammation, we have received generous research and creative assistance from a very gifted group of family, friends, and colleagues including the following: Grace Lau, RD, LD/N, CDE, a registered dietition and certified diabetes educator; Mindi Howell and Giny Wood for support and assistance; and James Russell, MS for the medical graphic art.

We especially want to express our sincerest gratitude to Chef Virginia McIlwain, a graduate of Le Cordon Bleu Academy, for her creativity and professional expertise used in creating the Pain-Free Recipes detailed in this program. Virginia will be adding new recipes regularly to our Web site at *www.painfreediet.com*, using the anti-inflammatory foods discussed in this book. We are extremely proud of Virginia and are so grateful for her contributions to this book.

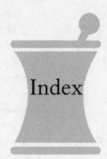

Index